D1266311

Pretty Pretty

Birth at home

Dedicated to
CHLOE FISHER
and
THE OXFORD COMMUNITY MIDWIVES
with admiration for the valuable work
they are doing for mothers,
babies, and families

Birth
at
home

BY

SHEILA KITZINGER

With Photographs by
SUZANNE ARMS

OXFORD
OXFORD UNIVERSITY PRESS
NEW YORK MELBOURNE
1979

Oxford University Press, Walton Street, Oxford OX2 6DP

OXFORD LONDON GLASGOW
NEW YORK TORONTO MELBOURNE WELLINGTON
IBADAN NAIROBI DAR ES SALAAM LUSAKA CAPE TOWN
KUALA LUMPUR SINGAPORE JAKARTA HONG KONG TOKYO
DELHI BOMBAY CALCUTTA MADRAS KARACHI

British Library Cataloguing in Publication Data

Kitzinger, Sheila
Birth at home. – (Oxford medical publications).
1. Childbirth at home
I. Title   II. Series
618.4   RG652   79-40149

ISBN 0-19-261160-7

Typeset by Visual Art Productions Ltd., Oxford
Printed in Great Britain
by R. Clay & Co., Ltd., Bungay

Acknowledgements

I particularly want to thank Suzanne Arms, the American photo-journalist, for her beautiful photographs and I am very grateful to her for her readiness to give ones which exactly match the mood of what I am trying to say about the special quality of a home birth which can celebrate a couple's love and caring for each other and the bonds uniting the family.

Thank you, Uwe, for your love and support and our daughters for understanding the importance of this work for me.

It sounds trite to say that this book would never have been written without my secretary Audrey Macefield, but it quite clearly would not. She is the perfect secretary!

The Manor   S.K.
Standlake
Oxon.
January 1979

A note to the reader: I refer to the baby as 'he' simply to distinguish the child from the mother.

Contents

1

Why birth at home
in the modern world?

'WHY anyone should want to write a book about birth at home nowadays is beyond me', the obstetrician said. 'I shouldn't think any woman would want to take the risk for her child. You ought to concentrate your efforts on making hospitals *more like home.*'

He has a point. It does look as if home birth is an anachronism in an age of increasing obstetric specialization and sophisticated (and expensive) technology. It is a matter that weighs heavily on a woman's mind in assessing the advantages and disadvantages of different places of birth not only for herself but for her baby. And there is a strong and irrefutable case for working to improve our maternity hospitals so that they are welcoming, friendly, comfortable places where the woman having a baby can relax and *be herself* and where maternity care is truly family centred. My *Good birth guide*[1] focuses on the conditions in hospitals seen mainly from mothers' points of view and is designed to help expectant parents know what questions to ask about policy and care, and changes that might be made in the hospitals to meet parents concerns.

Yet there are also very good reasons for writing about home birth in the West today and discussing why a woman may choose to give birth in her own home. Any system can be improved only when there are *alternatives* to that system. We can radically improve our culture of childbirth only when parents have choice about care and the setting in which they want to give birth.

The skills of arranging and conducting birth at home can quickly be forgotten in a society which directs all its attention to the organization of institutional deliveries. Bringing birth back into the home does not mean conveying the delivery suite technology and

[1] Fontana, London (1979).

1

atmosphere into the home. So it is also important to focus on planning for a home birth and how it can be arranged by all those sharing the experience in a spirit of joy and festivity.

This may sound rather too much to claim for birth at home. Maybe it would be wiser to concentrate simply on avoiding muddle and distress. But an important aspect of home birth is that it takes place in the environment which the couple have created together, and that it is here that there is the best chance of birth being celebrated as a natural part and a high point of the rhythm of their lives together. Although it is not impossible to create such an atmosphere in hospital, it is difficult and needs the concerted efforts of all concerned, from the hospital porter to the senior obstetrician, to make it like this. There are few hospitals which regularly build this atmosphere and those women who find it usually do so as a result of happy chance or their own tenacity in insisting that their labours are what they want them to be.

Birth at home is a birthday, a festive ritual as well as a physiological process. Bringing new life into the world has always been one of the great acts with symbolic significance beyond the task of pushing an infant out of a female body. Birth represents the creation of the new, the unfolding of fresh hope, the possibility of transmutation of everything that is old and faded into a world which is clean and lovely. Birth has also given us the concept of *rebirth,* the recreation of the human spirit, the purification of dross, the unsealing of eyes and ears so that the world is perceived in a new way. In all religions, from the simplest to the most complex, the concepts of birth and death, the beginning and the end, are integral to their understanding of the meaning of life.

In many ways in the West we have lost this awareness of themes of birth and death throughout life. We have turned childbirth and dying into medical conditions which are intended to take place outside the home in special institutions where they are managed by professionals who are not emotionally involved. Yet birth and death are the two things we must all inevitably confront. They are part of the ebb and flow of life itself. Perhaps we ought to ask how these universal human experiences can have meaning for us all. Only when basic human experiences like these have significance can we feel that we are creators instead of merely being at the mercy of fate, or of doctors, the 'them' who do things to us, and helpless in the cats' paws of large hierarchical organizations.

Why birth at home in the modern world?

This is why we need to 'demedicalize' birth and death. When medicine cannot help us, or when its techniques do not balance up with the *human* advantages to be gained from employing them, we must have the choice of saying 'no'. But if we are to have the opportunity of doing this we have to create alternatives in a society which is impoverished because in spite of the twentieth-century emphasis on freedom it offers most people little opportunity for any personal decision-making in health care.

We have to educate ourselves to make decisions. We need to learn the facts, the viable alternatives, the probable short- and long-term consequences and side-effects of our actions. We need to be able to stand at different vantage points and draw on all the information which experts can give us. But *we* have to make the decisions about health care, about the way in which we give birth, and so far as possible the way in which we pass through old age and die. To surrender these choices because professionals 'know best' is to surrender responsibility for our own lives.

This means creating a new kind of relationship with the medical profession, one in which doctors learn how to be educators. It is a joint enterprise. It is not just a question of new methods of providing health care, but of new attitudes.

Nowhere is this more important than in women's health care. Most doctors are men. Yet they have taken on responsibility for the health of the reproducers, women. In the USA gynaecologists have claimed the right to be the custodians of women's health *vis-à-vis* government. Yet they really know very little about it. They know about *disease*. It has never given a doctor much social esteem to describe himself as 'an obstetrician'. The gynaecologist, on the other hand, has relatively high status, obstetrics being just a sideline. Gynaecology is primarily concerned with surgery and endocrinology. Women do not need gynaecologists unless they are ill. But they have to have obstetricians when they have babies although they may be perfectly healthy.

It is only too easy for obstetricians to approach childbirth as if it, too, were a disease from which their expert knowledge is to cure women. The treatment of pregnancy and birth as pathological conditions leads to unnecessary and sometimes very harmful intervention in a natural process for which women's bodies are designed. The result is iatrogenic, or doctor-produced, illness which in turn calls for more intervention. The more iatrogenic

3

malfunction that is produced, the more necessary do doctors seem.

This is why it is important for women to learn about their bodies and how they function, and to know what doctors are talking about and the language in which the female body is described medically. But women need to go even further than this; they must get on good terms with their bodies, understanding them in a way for which technical information is only a beginning. The body is one's companion through life. One might as well make it a partner, rather than an enemy. A woman's body is a constantly changing companion too, passing through strange changes of shape, size, weight, and sensation as she reaches adolescence, experiences the cycles of menstruation with their effects on her body, closed or open, fluid-retaining and blood flowing, and changing even more dramatically through the reproductive cycle, in pregnancy and childbirth, and post-partum.

Obstetricians and gynaecologists know about this, but they usually do not live with the experience. It is to them a relatively unimportant matter compared with pathological conditions like cervical cancer or blocked Fallopian tubes. Yet it may be that carefully observing the body instead of trying to ignore it, understanding how to work with it throughout these natural cycles rather than fighting it, can often prevent the development of malfunction and resulting pathological conditions.

The home-birth movement which is now powerful in the United States and growing stronger in Britain is part of this larger movement to reassess the place of medicine in our lives, to create a new working relationship with doctors, and to accept responsibility for our own bodies.

2

What's wrong with
our hospitals?

ONE of the reasons why some women want to give birth at home is that many hospitals are not good enough. They are not good enough to provide an environment suited for a peak experience of one's life, nor for the birth of a family. But more than this, they are sometimes frankly dangerous places in which to have a baby.

In this chapter we shall be looking at some of the defects of the hospital environment, not with the intention of shocking or worrying expectant mothers, but with the premise that before things can be changed for the better, the consumers of care have a right to know the realities of obstetric practices and what goes on in hospitals. Some doctors believe that expectant mothers need protecting and that the really important thing is that they should trust the staff looking after them. But there has been sufficient public discussion about our health services today to make every pregnant woman aware that she must be prepared to ask for and if necessary insist on what she wants and must be an active not a passive partner in her own health care.

Moreover, men are less likely than women to see the advantages of home and the disadvantages of hospital. Women who are determined to have a home delivery sometimes have a hard time convincing their husbands, who feel that nothing can go really wrong in hospital and that it is the correct place in which to handle any medical crisis, of which childbirth is one. This chapter, therefore, is also written for those husbands who would prefer their wives to go into hospital.

The women's movement has emphasized that it is the responsibility of women to learn about how their bodies work and to demand full explanations concerning and choices in health care. This is not a responsibility we can abrogate during pregnancy simply by having faith in doctors. If we have a car accident or a heart attack we would be justified in accepting without question whatever help was offered in the emergency, but childbirth is a normal physiological function, an expression of health rather than a pathological condition.

It is sometimes taken for granted that any hospital is safer than any home. This is an entirely false assumption. There are excellent hospitals where a high-risk baby has the greatest chance of being born safely, but there are others which are badly staffed, poorly equipped, haphazardly run, in which the progress of labour is inadequately observed and the woman is left for long periods during which no one is aware of what is happening to her. There are hospitals in which a high-risk baby is at accentuated risk because there is no paediatrician or equipment for resuscitating a newborn who is not breathing, but because the birth takes place in hospital everyone is lulled into complacency. Outlying General Practitioner Units, although homely in atmosphere, are those most open to criticism in this respect, and women should only have their babies in these hospitals if everything is likely to be straightforward. (These women might also choose to have their babies at home.) Some general District Hospitals are also far away from a special-care baby-unit so that a baby needing special care has to be moved by ambulance and may be in a different hospital from its mother.

There are many hospitals in which routine procedures substitute for personal care. As a result women get induced when they go 10 days, 1 week, or even a few days over the estimated date of delivery, and receive standard doses of pethidine or other drugs regardless of whether they wish to have or need them; standard enemas or suppositories when they go into labour; perineal shaves; episiotomies before delivery, sleeping pills and laxatives afterwards; and where they have to conform to ward routines and feed their babies at times convenient to the staff. All this is not just a matter of irritation for the mother. When care is not adapted to personal needs it sometimes introduces additional and unnecessary risks for her and her baby.

This standardization is in large part the direct consequence of the organization of large-scale hierarchical institutions in which it is difficult to give much time or consideration to people as individuals, in which women are processed into becoming 'patients', and the patient population is subdivided into convenient

What's wrong with our hospitals?

categories, 'elderly primips', 'Caesars', 'multips', 'para 1s', and 'para 2s', or according to the consultants whose beds they are in. Sometimes women having babies are described under the generic heading of 'mothers', 'mums', or 'girls'. In some hospitals a woman's personal identity seems to be recognized only by the plastic tag fixed round her wrist indicating who she is.

In hospital the territory is quite clearly under the control of the staff, not the women having babies in it. Whereas when a baby is born at home the midwife and doctor are guests, in hospital they are in charge. There are rules and regulations to which patients must conform, some clearly stated and obvious to all, others unwritten and difficult to discover until they have been violated. Part of the task of learning how to be a good patient in hospital is finding out what these are from other patients so that one can conform to the nurses' and doctors' expectations. In some maternity hospitals a 'sixth-form dorm' atmosphere develops, which some women quite enjoy, as they co-operate in showing each other 'the ropes', in covering for each other in doing things which are disapproved of by nurses (such as having a bath at the wrong time or feeding a baby during visiting hours) and share the same kind of impersonal autocratic treatment.

Much of what passes for childbirth education today in the United States is instruction to help women face the challenge of being in the alien environment of a hospital, to learn how to be tactful and 'sensible' in their requests and tolerate with equanimity the many assaults on the person which are a standard part of obstetric care. Lee Stewart, the co-founder of NAPSAC (National Association of Parents and Professionals for Safe Alternatives in Childbirth) asks childbirth educators: 'Have you . . . ever stopped to think how much class time is spent teaching couples to cope with hospitals instead of . . . teaching about the birth process?'[1] It seems a fair question, and many antenatal teachers are spending more and more time explaining the modern technology of obstetrics rather than helping women get to understand their own bodies better and to prepare themselves for the physiological and psychological adventure of labour.

But at least maternity patients have a defined place in the hospital. The fathers of the babies may find themselves in a kind of

[1] Lee Stewart: Why is there a need for alternatives in childbirth? In *Safe alternatives in childbirth* (ed. David and Lee Stewart). NAPSAC, Chapel Hill (1976)

7

limbo, allowed in but not welcomed, and without advance notice, at any moment ejected. The claim has been made that expectant fathers in our society are 'culturally submerged' and that although increasing numbers are present in the delivery wards they are given only 'token recognition', often as unpaid comforters to alleviate staff shortages.[1] Their presence is usually considered neither necessary nor desirable by hospital staff during admission procedures when the women is 'prepped' and they are almost invariably asked to wait outside. Richman and Goldthorp remark that the man then undergoes an 'entrance trauma' as his wife is taken away from him by a midwife who treats him as a 'non-person'. When at last he is told that he can come in he must put on sterile garments, emphasizing that 'he is in a culturally alien environment as a dependant'. In gown, mask, cap, and overshoes he becomes ostensibly part of the medical team. In reality, however, he is 'at the lowest level of involvement', has no recognized responsibility and often feels that he is there on sufferance. He may not know where to stand, what he is allowed to do, or even whether it is all right to touch his wife. Certain parts of the delivery room are the private territories of the staff,[2] but they are not publicly demarcated so he cannot know when he is in danger of invading them. He is surrounded by gleaming machinery and instruments, the purpose of which he does not understand and which look forbidding. This equipment may physically separate him from his wife and he may be reluctant to ask whether it is all right to go to the other side of the bed or move the monitor a few inches so that he can get close to her. Once the second stage begins, everyone around him is masked, so he may not even be able to tell from expressions on people's faces whether he is conducting himself correctly.

In many hospitals in which the father is permitted to be present during labour and at delivery there are occasions on which he is told to leave, and after some of these he may not be asked to come in again, either because his presence is not thought desirable or because staff have forgotten he was there. Some couples dread being separated in this arbitrary manner; the man feels unnecessary

[1] Joel Richman and G. O. Goldthorp: Fatherhood, the social construction of pregnancy and birth. In *The place of birth* (ed. Sheila Kitzinger and John Davis). Oxford University Press (1978).
[2] Richman and Goldthorp in *The place of birth,* op. cit.

and unwanted and the woman is deprived of emotional support from her husband when she needs it most. The times when the husband is told to wait outside are mainly those in which examinations are performed and obstetric manoeuvres done, and when progress or failure to progress is assessed and plans are made for intervening in labour, setting up drips and giving analgesia or anaesthesia. In some hospitals the arrival of a consultant on the scene heralds the request for the man to wait outside the room while the obstetrician examines the patient. A woman has to be very alert and self-confident to be quick enough to say to the obstetrician, 'Oh, do please let my husband stay. I should so much like it if he were here', or something of the kind, and even then the obstetrician may feel embarrassed about doing a vaginal examination on a woman in her husband's presence.

Men often say that they have been allowed to come back into the room only to discover that their wives have received drugs which they had asked beforehand not to have, narcotics which are given by injection being the main culprits here, or have agreed to have an epidural because they have been told that there is slow progress and 'it is going to get much worse'.

Sometimes labour has been accelerated by an intravenous drip of oxytocin without the labouring woman having had a chance to discuss this, and occasionally without her knowledge (this can happen when she is told that she is being given intravenous glucose; the first bottle set up usually is a glucose solution; after that has begun to drip into her bloodstream Syntocin is set up as well).

But in some units husbands are also asked to go out for other minor procedures where they would be unlikely to affect any member of staff's judgement by causing embarrassment. Examples are when the woman uses a bedpan, when the midwife palpates the abdomen to find out the position of the baby, or even sometimes when blood pressure is checked. In hospitals where this fragmenting of the continuity of the relationship between the couple occurs the husband may be on tenterhooks all the time, not knowing when he will be sent out next, and the woman has no one on whom she can rely for constant emotional support.

Many obstetricians are unwilling to do a forceps delivery in the presence of the husband, even though the same obstetricians insist that 'lift out' forceps are simple to use and the labour is still 'natural'. Some obstetricians believe that because it would cut down the length of the second stage of labour much trauma could be saved the mother's perineal tissues and the baby's head if most babies were lifted out between steel blades in this way. One head of obstetrics in a busy university hospital told me that he had been convinced by his experience in Boston, Massachusetts, and his observation of the proportion of forceps deliveries done there, that induction of multigravidae at term along with lift-out forceps at delivery was the best way to have a baby. Since husbands are frequently turned out for forceps deliveries this means that in spite of hospital policies to admit husbands and the increasing numbers of men who now want to be present, in those hospitals where these obstetric policies are followed more men are now not being permitted to see the birth of their babies.

Richman and Goldthorp[1] found that fathers who were present at delivery, not only during labour, tended to feel more positive about the whole experience than fathers who had gone out once delivery was imminent. Fifty per cent of those men who were at the delivery thought their wives had had a 'comfortable' time, whereas 52 per cent of those attending the labour only thought their wives had had a 'difficult' time. Perhaps this is why they went out. But it does suggest that being outside the room, not knowing what is going on inside, may let some men's fantasies of pain and injury run away with them, so that the labour becomes an ordeal for *them*. It is possible that those who wanted to be present for delivery had had better previous preparation about what was happening and how they could help than those who wished to be there for the labour only, and that wanting to be there at the birth was a reflection of better education about the whole process. Good preparation of fathers is an important part of the care and welcome which hospitals should provide, and this is frequently lacking. In most hospitals classes in preparation for childbirth include one, or at most two, evenings for expectant fathers, where they tend to be given only the most rudimentary information.

When fathers were asked what they liked about the labour and delivery 53 per cent of those attending the birth stressed the wonder and beauty of the delivery itself. Among both the birth attenders and those who were present during labour only, the chance to support their wives was emphasized as an experience which gave

[1] In *The place of birth,* op. cit.

them satisfacton. Richman and Goldthorp comment that men expressed themselves in terms which are 'normally associated with femininity . . . the first sight of the baby's head was beautiful; it was a joy seeing the first start of life; the happiness of nine months coming to fruition'. When fathers are made to leave before the delivery they are deprived of a very positive experience.

The time immediately following birth may be as important as the birth itself in terms of the relationship between the couple and between father, mother, and baby. Although there is increasing concern in hospitals about the provision of an environment which is suitable for bonding between mother and baby, the importance of bonding between *father* and baby is not always recognized and the conditions in which it can occur are often absent. In some units the father does not usually hold his baby; after the mother has held (sometimes only touched) it the infant is put in a perspex crib where it can be admired from afar. In some hospitals, too, husbands are bundled away shortly after delivery, instead of being allowed time alone with wife and baby to get to know each other as a family. Although it is the custom in many units to give husband and wife a cup of tea together, once this ceremony has been performed it may be suggested that it is an appropriate time for the man to leave.

In hospital most women need suturing of the perineum because they have had episiotomies. Episiotomy occurs so frequently today that it is considered a normal and in some units inevitable and necessary part of childbirth. In many hospitals it appears to be used more or less routinely with all primigravidae, unless they deliver extraordinarily easily and speedily. Husbands are often asked to leave before the stitching, and for some women this is the most painful part of childbirth because it is done inexpertly and sometimes roughly, and without adequate anaesthetization of the perineal tissues.

Thus at the time when the new family is born, and when the couple might be focusing pleasurably on the new life they have together created, the parents are separated from each other and the baby, and the woman is subjected to the endurance test of examination and suturing of the perineum.

In my own study of some British maternity hospitals[1] there was a time after this too, when some women said they missed their

---

[1] *The good birth guide,* Fontana, London (1979).

husbands. Although in some units the man is allowed to go with his wife and baby to the ward and to sit with her, in many the admission of the woman to the postpartum ward is the signal for a parting of the ways, the man being sent home and the baby often going to the nursery, even if it has not already been sent there. Women often said that they passed sleepless hours excitedly re-living the experience through which they had passed, longing for their husbands and their babies, lying alone behind drawn curtains or in the dark, afraid of disturbing other mothers or being 'a nuisance' on the ward. Those women who had difficult labours often seemed to need to make sense of their experiences, especially if they felt that they had in some way 'failed'. If they had been heavily drugged there were often large sections of labour which they could not remember or which did not fit into the pattern of the whole, and they wanted to talk it through and discover when and why different things had occurred and been done to them. The husband who had been present was the obvious person with which to do this, and yet he had been sent away.

From the man's point of view, separation following childbirth may leave him feeling isolated and, after he has rung up relatives and made the glad announcement to as many people as he can, strangely depressed.

The new father usually rings the antenatal teacher to tell her of the birth. With those couples I have taught I always ask the man how *he* is feeling. The answers are sometimes surprising. When babies have been born at home fathers always express positive emotions, but when a man has had to leave his wife in hospital and has come home to the empty house, no longer needed, he often says that he is feeling depressed or 'low'; he usually expresses this initially in terms of 'tiredness' or 'exhaustion' partly because he does not feel that depression is justified. But when we discuss his feelings further he reveals that there is a profound sense of being *unwanted*. When a man has experienced the birth as a peak experience the contrast between his wife's dependence on him then and her obvious need of him in labour and his postpartum loneliness and isolation is often marked. Postnatal depression and the third and fourth day 'blues' are wellknown, though little understood, maternal experiences. Far less is known of the *father's* postnatal depression, one which he may feel it unmanly to reveal in any way. Probably in most men the aetiology of this depression is

12

entirely social; it is a direct consequence of hospital birth and the subsequent separation of the husband and father from his wife and new-born child. Such depression may have little effect on the relationship between husband and wife, but it is possible that it contributes to some women's difficulties in postpartum emotional adjustment and their adaptation to the new and challenging tasks of motherhood.

Hospitals will only offer an environment for birth in which this immediate postpartum period is also made a positive experience for both parents when they provide double beds large enough to accommodate husband, wife, and new baby together. This is already being done in one hospital in California. I cannot envisage some British hospitals taking to it with alacrity.

In another study of 65 women who sought to have their babies at home[1] I discovered that they often do so because they wish to avoid the interventionist practices of modern obstetrics, preferring to trust in nature unless it is clear that other help is needed. One of the obstetric practices questioned by many women is induction of labour for social and administrative or for minor medical reasons. They have good reason to criticize the use of any medical procedures for *non*-medical reasons and especially to question the use of induction for social purposes or trivial medical reasons, not only from the point of view of their own comfort and well-being, but also from that of the baby's safety. For elective induction can be dangerous, mainly by reducing the amount of oxygen available to the baby and by producing extreme pressure on its head.

In an American study in which foetal heart rhythms in spontaneous labours and others which were induced for social reasons were compared, it was found that there was a much higher incidence of deceleration in the foetal heart rate 'due to greater intensity of contractions and counterpressure on the foetal head caused by greater resistance of the birth canal'.[2] Most of these type-1 dips are harmless and many of the babies are delivered with no problems at all, but it has been suggested that sometimes these dips are associated with 'uneven compression and deformation of

---

[1] Sheila Kitzinger and John Davis (Eds.): *The place of birth,* Oxford University Press (1978).
[2] Ricardo L. Schwartz *et al.*: Fetal and maternal monitoring in spontaneous labors and elective inductions. *American Journal of Obstetrics and Gynecology* **120,** 356 – 62 (1974).

the foetal head with EEG alterations, cerebral lesions and neurologic sequelae'. Probably most mothers would consider that this is a risk not worth taking and it is clear that a great many of those who sought home birth would have required compelling reasons for agreeing to induction of labour.

Some of these women choosing to have babies at home have had previous induced labours, often without full discussion, and want the next labour to be as natural as possible. They often feel that the labour was unnecessarily painful,[1] hurried, and generally stressful, and had the experience of being separated from their babies who had to go for observation to the nursery following delivery.

But it is not just a question of women's feelings. Induction of labour always carries some risk for mother and baby because there is no standard safe dose of oxytocin. The only way of finding out what a particular uterus and a particular foetus can tolerate is by dripping in oxytocin and seeing what happens. Uterine sensitivity to oxytocin is very variable and where one woman may require only 2 milliunits to get labour going another may need as much as 30 milliunits. One advocate of active management warns that 'if too much oxytocin is used and hyperstimulation occurs, there will be a gradual prolongation of the contractions, an increase in their frequency and a rise in the resting tone of the uterus [its muscle tone between contractions]. These changes may result in statis of blood in the intravillous space and may eventually lead to foetal anoxia'[2] [i.e. the baby is short of oxygen]. This is why careful observation and continuous monitoring of the foetus and contractions is so important when labour is induced. When intravenous oxytocin is used combined with amniotomy [rupturing of the membranes] there are 3 times as many babies who have difficulty in breathing at birth than when labour is not induced.[3] Labour may sometimes have been induced *because* the baby was not in a good state, but such respiratory depression in babies is directly related to the *amount* of oxytocin given.[4]

[1] *Some mothers' experience of induced labour* (2nd edn). The National Childbirth Trust, London (1978).
[2] Ian Brown: Active management of labour. *Midwife and Health Visitor* 9, July (1973).
[3] R. Chamberlain (Ed.): *British births 1970,* Vol. I: *The first week of life.* Heinemann, London (1975).
[4] W. A. Liston and A. J. Campbell: Danger of oxytocin-induced labour to foetuses. *British Medical Journal* iii, 606 – 7 (1974).

What's wrong with our hospitals?

Many obstetricians nowadays believe in 'the active management of labour' and see their task as one of ensuring that dilatation takes place progressively and within a defined length of time without waiting to see what happens if things are left to nature or retrospective diagnosis of prolonged labour is made. The partogram, a statistical curve of the average rate of effacement and dilatation of the cervix and descent of the presenting part, has become the norm against which individual labour is measured. It is a good guide, but perhaps a bad master. Regardless of how the mother is feeling or the strength of her contractions at present, if the curve of her labour is to the left of the normal curve a drip is set up and labour is augmented with oxytocin. The obstetrician's aim is to get each woman delivered within 24 hours, 12 hours, or 8 hours, depending on his personal philosophy. Everything else is considered abnormal.

The length of any labour is to some extent, however, a subjective evaluation and depends on when the woman decides to go into hospital or notices that she is having regular contractions, and on when the first vaginal examination is made to measure dilatation. Labour can only be said to be occurring when there is evidence of some dilatation of the cervix. Yet many women start labour already partially dilated, often by 2 centimetres or so, sometimes by 3 or 4 centimetres, and occasionally by more, because of effective pre-labour contractions which have occurred in the immediately preceding days and weeks, so even this measurement is imprecise. The precise timing of labour may give a sense of security to those managing it but is in most cases a will-o'-the-wisp of the obstetric imagination. There is no reason to think that rapid labours are safer or longer labours are more dangerous for the baby. The British Births Survey[1] showed that no more babies died with prolonged labours where delivery eventually occurred spontaneously than with short labours, although where forceps were used in delivery the risk to the baby was increased.

My study of women's experiences in 300 British hospitals[2] indicated that although women were often asked what they thought about induction of labour and were able to discuss its pros and cons, they were hardly ever consulted about acceleration of labour

[1] G. Chamberlain, E. Philipp, B. Howlet, and K. Masters: *British births 1970*, Vol. II *Obstetric care*. Heinemann, London (1978).
[2] *The place of birth,* op. cit.

by oxytocin drip. They were the passive recipients of care and from this point had to hand over to the obstetrician control of their own bodies.

This happened because obstetric intervention, of whatever kind, unless wisely and discreetly employed, tends to produce a situation in which further intervention is required. It is a self-perpetuating system. Making contractions stronger, longer, and more frequent with a Syntocin drip is likely to increase the pain of labour, sometimes very suddenly, so that the woman feels unable to cope with contractions and asks for pain relief. Since this is well known, the woman is often advised to have drugs for pain relief before or just after the drip is set up. She may be told that she is bound to need it, so she might as well have it now before things get 'too bad'.

She may be offered pethidine, still the most widely used analgesic drug in Britain. This is given by injection in doses of up to 200 milligrams. Its disadvantages are two-fold: the woman becomes drowsy, sometimes nauseated, sometimes hallucinated, and is less likely to organize and control her response to pain than before she received it; and the baby is affected because all drugs put into the mother's bloodstream travel through the placenta and umbilical cord into the foetus, who is far less able to tolerate massive doses of a hard drug even than its mother, and who is delivered in a doped condition. Pethidine is available for home births as well as those in hospitals, but tends to be given in much smaller doses when it is used. Whereas at home a woman may receive 100 milligrams at most, and often does not need any at all, frequently in hospitals today she is given doses of 150 milligrams and these are repeated every few hours, so that many women are receiving 500 milligrams of pethidine before delivery.[1] Sometimes the effect of pethidine is to slow down labour. So a synthetic hormone has been introduced into a woman's bloodstream to augment a labour and because of the effects of this she has been given a drug which reduces the efficiency of uterine action, so that the drip has to be adjusted to a faster rate to ensure that the uterus continues to contract, thus producing more pain. It is a vicious circle.

This does not happen when regional anaesthesia is given because pain can thereby be completely removed. This accounts for the popularity of epidurals. But the very fact that a woman can feel

[1] K. O'Driscoll: An obstetrician's view of pain. *British Journal of Anaesthesia* **47**, 1053 (1975).

nothing means that violence can be done to her uterus without her ever being aware of it. Staff must observe carefully to guard against the risks of uterine rupture, for when labour is accelerated and contractions are powerful, long-lasting and rapidly recurring there is a danger that the uterus cannot stand the strain and that the muscle wall tears. There are other risks when an epidural is given: that the anaesthesia may be introduced into the spinal cavity instead of the epidural space so that a full spinal anaesthetic is given, with the likely consequence of a post-spinal headache which may last for days or sometimes even weeks and be the worst headache a woman has ever known; that an epidural given inexpertly may anaesthetize the mother's breathing apparatus, so that an antidote must be quickly given to allow her to breathe freely (a rare, but nevertheless possible, occurrence); that the mother's blood-pressure suddenly drops and that blood flow to the baby is reduced (this is often only a temporary effect, lasting 10 minutes or so, but may make the woman feel faint, giddy and sick, and sometimes results in unconsciousness); that the epidural only 'takes' one side, so that the mother has to handle one-sided contractions, which many experience as especially painful perhaps because they anticipated full pain relief. An expected consequence of an epidural is that the woman is no longer aware of the need to empty her bladder and cannot do so that a catheter must be introduced, thus increasing the chances of pelvic infection. Bladder function may be affected for some hours, and occasionally longer, after delivery. Another very rare consequence of an epidural is paraplegia, the woman never recovering the use of her legs. Although this is extremely unlikely to happen, every doctor needs to remain aware of the danger of regional anaesthesia and epidurals should never be done casually.

Under the circumstances it is hardly surprising that some women are willing to forgo the undoubted advantages of an epidural in a labour which is difficult or painful and choose to give birth in a place where it is impossible to give an epidural at all, believing that although the analgesic effect of concentrating on, say, a bunch of daises in a mug on the dressing table or breathing one's way through contractions may not be so great as that of an epidural, it is unquestionably safer.

Another practice involved in the active management of labour is amniotomy or artificial rupture of the membranes. This is so often

Birth at home

done when the woman is admitted to hospital provided that there is sufficient dilatation (about 3 centimetres) to reach the membranes easily. It is a painless operation and not one that need cause anxiety in terms of the mother's sensations, but it is a practice which is open to criticism on several counts. For while the membranes are still intact the foetus is an aquatic creature, moving relatively freely in water. Once they have ruptured, whether spontaneously or artificially, contractions can cause compression on the cord, which carries oxygen-saturated blood to the foetus, and as the presenting part is pressed down into the cervix and through the pelvic outlet, also lead to marked moulding of the baby's head.[1] Moreover, once the membranes have ruptured pelvic infection can occur if the woman has not delivered within a reasonable period of time (24 hours is often considered the limit) and a forceps delivery is carried out, or a Caesarean section if the cervix is not adequately dilated, once the time limit is reached. There would therefore seem to be a case for leaving the membranes intact as long as possible. Obstetricians, however, use the condition of the liquor in which the baby floats as a diagnostic tool. If it contains meconium, the contents of the foetal intestines, the foetus may be distressed. One argument for rupturing the membranes is that it allows the obstetrician to observe the amniotic fluid. (The only other way of observing this is with an amnioscope, a small light introduced through the cervix which can reveal the state of the fluid inside the intact membranes. Few obstetricians use these.)

Once the membranes have ruptured the presenting part is pressed firmly through the cervix, and this has the effect of intensifying contractions. It is one way, therefore, in which labour can be speeded up and contractions made more efficient. But there is a still more powerful reason why amniotomy is performed increasingly at an early phase of labour, and this is because once it is done an electrode or 'clip' can be inserted into the foetal scalp to record heartbeats and the obstetrician can know much more accurately the state of the foetus. It gives, in effect, a window into the womb. Of course once the heartbeats are recorded the meaning of different rates and rhythms has to be interpreted. The foetal heart rate normally slows a little at the height of strong contractions but should

[1] Roberto Caldeyro-Barcia: Some consequences of obstetrical interference. *Birth and the Family Journal* 2, 34 – 76, (1975).

pick up again once the contraction is finished. This particular form of intervention is employed therefore to give the obstetrician more accurate information, in particular when induction or acceleration is being used—another instance of one kind of intervention requiring another. A woman who believes strongly that the membranes should be left intact unless there is a strong reason for rupturing them may find it difficult to get concessions from obstetricians in hospital so that she can labour on without amniotomy. At home she is much more likely to be allowed to wait till the waters burst by themselves. (This may happen during a vaginal examination when the membranes are bulging, even though the midwife did not intend to do an artificial rupture.)

One effect of many kinds of obstetric intervention in labour is that the mother must stay in bed and is more or less immobilised. This can increase discomfort, and is associated with contractions which are less effective than contractions when the woman is standing and walking about although they are more painful.[1,2,3]

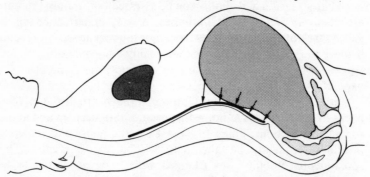

FIG. 1. In late pregnancy women have an exaggerated sacro-lumbar curve and ordinary chairs do not give enough support. This is why a couple of pillows are inadequate for labour and specially adapted back support can make for much greater comfort

Lying supine, flat on the bed on one's back, causes pressure on the inferior vena cava, one of the main blood vessels, which when lying beneath the heavy uterus has a restricted blood flow (Fig. 1). It

[1] A. Flynn and J. Kelly: Continuous fetal monitoring in the ambulant patient in labour. *British Medical Journal* ii, 842 – 3 (1976).

[2] N. Smyth: Biomechanics and human parturition. *Proceedings of the Royal Society of Medicine* 67, 189 – 93 (1974).

[3] Gertie F. Marx: Aortocaval compression. *Bulletin of the New York Academy of Medicine* 50, 443 – 6 (1974).

results in hypotension (low blood-pressure) in the mother, sometimes palpitations and even unconsciousness, and a reduced flow of oxygenated blood to the foetus. This is why women are now encouraged to lie on their sides when in labour and why even when a Caesarean section is performed it may be done with the mother's trunk tilted.

Walking about, if it is comfortable, is even better. A woman's body tells her soon enough when she should sit or crouch for the delivery. In one study [1] of women who were allowed to walk round compared with others who were kept in bed it was found that labour was shorter, the need for pain-relieving drugs less and the babies' heartbeats more regular in those who kept walking. A greater number of women in the group in bed had such long-drawn-out labours that doctors augmented labour with a Syntocin drip. Moreover, the babies of the mothers who had been walking about were in a better state after delivery and had higher Apgar scores at 1 and 5 minutes. (The Apgar score is a method by which the newborn baby's health and vitality can be assessed very simply 1 minute after delivery and again at 5 minutes. A baby in perfect condition gets a mark of 10. Most babies score 7 or more. The second reading is more important than the first and many who start off with low Apgar scores at 1 minute have one of 9 or 10 at 5 minutes. See page 21.)

Until recently women in hospital were *expected* to lie flat on their backs in bed, whereas at home they would have been up and about for much of labour, doing small tasks in the house and changing position frequently in the natural course of events. This spontaneous mobility was changed when women started to be admitted to hospital, perhaps only because it is part of the expectation of behaviour of hospital patients that they should lie in bed, and it was not until adverse effects were noted and research done which indicated that the supine position was deleterious that customs were changed. One wonders how many other apparently minor, subtle modifications of behaviour occur because a woman is in hospital instead of at home and what further harmful effects of hospital customs remain to be discovered.

Some women who seek home birth are concerned about continuous foetal monitoring. They may be worried that

[1] A. M. Flynn, J. Kelly, G. Hollins, P. F. Lynch: Ambulation in labour, *British Medical Journal* **ii**, 591 – 3, 1978.

What's wrong with our hospitals?

The Apgar score

Symptom	The baby scores 2 if	The baby scores 1 if	The baby scores 0 if
Colour	Pink	Trunk is pink, hands and feet blue	Completely blue or grey
Pulse	100 or more per minute	Less than 100	Non-existent
Reflex response to tapping the soles of the feet	Crying	Just a change of facial expression	None
State of muscle tone shown by	Active movements	Slight movements	Limpness
Breathing	Vigorous with strong cry	Slow and irregular	Absent

immobility will have ill effects, be anxious that misinterpretation of the tracings by inexperienced doctors may lead to an unnecessary forceps delivery or Caesarean section, or be apprehensive about the machinery not working correctly or breaking down. Some query the humanity of screwing a miniature corkscrew metal attachment or a clip into an unborn baby's scalp. Since more and more mothers are being monitored as hospitals acquire the machine, and many obstetricians have a goal of 100-per-cent monitoring, women whose babies are in no way 'at risk' are being automatically given the treatment used on babies who are genuinely at risk and whose heart rhythms require careful watching.

A few mothers, too, are concerned lest their babies are left with a permanent bald patch on their heads where the electrode was introduced. This may seem a minor price to pay for having every heartbeat monitored, but one mother who was not at special risk, who was monitored against her wishes, and whose baby was affected in this way, commented during her second pregnancy that she felt very reluctant to submit herself to any more obstetric 'gadgetry'.

Birth at home

Women are also beginning to question the need for episiotomy (a cut in the perineal tissue and muscle layer to enlarge the vaginal opening), and some think they should be given the choice of whether or not to have one. At home midwives pride themselves on delivery with an intact perineum wherever possible, working with the mother so that delivery is gentle, and judging whether or not an episiotomy is necessary in that particular case and thus avoiding unnecessary interference.

A midwife commenting on her hospital experience says: 'it is an absolute disgrace on the midwife's part to allow a perineum to tear; even a small nick which requires no suturing is considered thoroughly inefficient', and adds that a young midwife or pupil is 'so terrified of allowing a perineum to tear that to do a routine episiotomy becomes the easiest answer. No one is ever criticised for an unnecessary episiotomy'.[1] Midwives and doctors thus never learn how to judge the state of the perineum or how to help mothers deliver without episiotomies.

It is this kind of thing that worries many women about delivering in hospital. They prefer to retain their own autonomy and to give birth as naturally as possible in their own homes.

Woman may also want to be assured that they will not be separated from their babies for any reason whatever, that they will be able to take them into their arms immediately following delivery and keep them beside them, if they wish in their beds, from that moment on. This is often difficult or impossible to arrange in hospital, and in some hospitals babies are arbitrarily removed from their mothers as if they belonged to the hospital rather than their parents.

Some women want to have home births because they have had the experience after a previous labour of having their babies taken away from them.[2] In some of these hospitals where there are special-care baby-units, especially if they are on the same floor of the building as the delivery rooms, cots in these units are somehow kept full or almost full, even when there are few sick on very underweight babies.[3]

But whether or not their babies were taken to special care, in one

[1] Dinah Levett: Some thoughts on episiotomies *N.C.T. Teachers' Broadsheet 22,* National Childbirth Trust, London, (1973).
[2] *The place of birth,* op. cit.
[3] *The good birth guide,* op. cit.

What's wrong with our hospitals?

study[1] of women whose labours had been induced 42 per cent were separated from their babies in the sense that they were unable to hold them or have time in which to get to know them, or if they had had this opportunity were unable to take advantage of it because they were too heavily drugged or could not remember afterwards that they had seen and perhaps touched their babies. Research by Klaus and Kennell in Cleveland[2] shows that seeing, hearing, touching, and exploring the newborn baby within minutes of delivery is the psychological mechanism by which bonding spontaneously occurs between mother and baby, and that separation may make it much harder for a mother to relate to her baby and to feel that it is really hers. Some mothers, writing to me some time after their reports of their experiences of induced labour had been sent to me, told how bonding had been delayed and of their difficulties in being able to mother their babies. A smaller group, writing when their babies were about one year old, indicated that this had had a prolonged effect on their relationship with their children, and a few of these women revealed that they had been battering their babies and used the chance to write about their experiences as a way of seeking help.

Frédérick Leboyer has drawn attention to the baby's experience of birth[3] and believes that we should examine the way in which we welcome babies into the world. He says that new-born babies have feelings and that they should not be treated as hunks of meat; in a 'paroxysm of confusion, of despair and distress . . . someone seizes the baby by a foot and lets it hang over the void.' He suggests that the room should be dimly lit, voices hushed, that whoever is delivering should allow the cord to stop pulsating before it is clamped and cut, and that the baby should be handled gently and be put in a warm bath a few minutes after birth.

Those couples who want Leboyer-style deliveries meet insuperable difficulties in hospitals where the Leboyer philosophy is not understood or where staff are in disagreement with his teachings. Even where hospitals state that they do Leboyer births this is variously interpreted.[4] It may mean, for example, gentle delivery, but immediate cutting of the cord, and attendants may be

[1] *Some mothers' experiences of induced labour,* op. cit.
[2] M. Klaus and J. Kennell: *Maternal infant bonding:* Mosby, St. Louis (1976).
[3] Frederick Leboyer: *Birth without violence.* Fontana, London (1977).
[4] *The good birth guide,* op. cit.

23

unwilling to forgo the routine of mucus extraction, although the result of stimulating the posterior pharynx of the new-born baby's larynx by inexpert use of a mucous catheter or suction tubing is laryngeal inhibition, so that the baby may not breathe and needs to be resuscitated. Obsessionally suctioning every drop of mucus can do more harm than good, but unfortunately this is what midwives and doctors are trained to do. In the great majority of hospitals it is not possible for the baby to be bathed as Leboyer recommends. For this reason too women may choose home birth so that they themselves can remain in charge and create the setting in which the baby can be welcomed in to life.

Women planning on a home birth who have had a previous baby in hospital often cite lack of opportunity to breastfeed as they wished to as a reason for choosing home birth. Of 74 accounts of hospital births by women choosing home birth, only 9 women felt entirely happy about the support and assistance they had with breastfeeding.[1] Mothers who intend to breastfeed and want to feed their babies whenever they ask are more likely than ever before to find a hospital in which they can feed on demand, but demand feeding is also subject to a wide range of interpretations in different units and by different staff within the same unit.[1,2] It often does not mean 'whenever the baby seems to want to suckle' but 'not more often than every 2 hours' or 'when it does not interrupt ward routine'.

Women who have babies in hospitals are not only separated from their husbands, at least overnight, and often for large sections of each day as well, but must also be away from their older children. Family life is interrupted and in some hospitals toddlers are still not allowed on the wards or to see the new baby.[3] There are some shining exceptions. I know of several hospitals where the older child is encouraged to climb into its mother's bed for a cuddle with the baby. But in other hospitals older siblings are treated as an unfortunate nuisance, their presence disturbing ward routines and interfering with mothers' rest. It is understandable that the arrival of numbers of 2 – 5-year-olds on a public ward should produce noise, excitement, laughter, and tears and that other women find it

[1] *The good birth guide*, op. cit.
[2] Sheila Kitzinger: *The experience of breastfeeding*. Penguin, Harmondsworth (1979).
[3] *The good birth guide*, op. cit.

impossible to sleep, read, or even talk quietly while this is going on. This is another reason why hospital may not be the best place after the baby is born and why the woman who already has children should consider either having her baby at home or being discharged from hospital within a few hours of the birth if possible.

It is an indictment of many of our maternity hospitals that women wanting home birth do so not only because of their positive attitude to home as a place of delivery but because they are anxious about what happens in hospitals and procedures which reduce their capacity to see themselves as effective and able to cope with their labours and their babies. Many of the things that concern these women about the new advanced technology and mechanization of birth, are those which obstetricians see as indications of advance in the management of labour. Others, attitudes to fathers and other children in many hospitals, for example, suggest that our hospitals are out of step with the times and are not in tune with the quality of relationships sought either between couples and in families or in the informed partnership which women want with their doctors. So on one hand there is evidence of sophisticated, technological control of labour, and on the other of anachronistic rules which regulate the behaviour of individuals within the hospital, inculcating in women a learned helplessness, and moulding them into compliant patients instead of active birth-givers and mothers able to take on responsibility for their babies from the moment of delivery.

It is only by creating alternatives to hospital that options can be kept open and that we can be aware of the possibility of other ways of birthing. Hospitals need to change but the direction in which they change is dependant on the existence of other models, other kinds of environment in which birth takes place. Without home births and the new ventures that are made there in the setting of different personal philosophies and life styles, the range of likely changes in hospital birth-styles is very limited; it tends to be the accumulation of new kinds of 'hardware', new techniques, new ways of 'managing' labour or mother and baby, rather than different attitudes and a new atmosphere.

The opportunity to have home births ensures that alternatives to the system remain, and that there is at least the possibility that as hospitals change they do so in such a way that they acquire some of the qualities of friendliness, intimacy, personal caring, and peace which are an integral part of birth at home.

3
Safety

EVERY woman having a baby at home should realize that there is a small, but nevertheless real, additional risk compared with birth in a well-equipped, well-run, and well-staffed hospital. Unforeseen emergencies can occur, even when everything has been apparently normal throughout pregnancy, which only a hospital can deal with. This is why it is unwise to choose home birth unless one is within an hour's distance of hospital. Some people would think one ought to be nearer still. This is a matter for discussion. There can be no hard and fast rules about it. The important thing is that the mother should feel safe and that she should herself decide on the degree of acceptable risk.

Statistical evidence directly relevant to the safety of different places of birth is very out of date. Fedrick and Butler[1] used material from the 1959 perinatal mortality study. Although it showed a slightly increased risk with home births in that year, the maternity services have undergone radical reorganization since then and midwifery training has changed considerably. We have no means of knowing whether birth at home has become safer or more risky, nor whether birth in hospital is safer or more dangerous than it was in 1958. There are still far more deaths in hospital than at home, but this might mean that mothers with high-risk factors are delivered in hospital as they should be. However, since home births are now rare, increasing numbers of mothers with no high-risk factors are having their babies in hospital and this must have an effect on the perinatal mortality risks. The question is whether the ratio of babies dying or taking a long time to take their first breath in hospital has been reduced sufficiently to justify the widely accepted conclusion that hospital provides greater safety for all babies than does birth at home.

[1] Jean Fedrick and R. O. Butler: Intended place of delivery and perinatal outcome. *British Medical Journal* i, 763 – 5 (1978).

Birth at home

We do not live always thinking in terms of risks, but take them all the time. Whenever we cross a road, light a gas stove, go swimming, travel by plane, there is an element of risk. Life would come to a standstill if we were incapable of taking risks. In many of these situations we must rely on other, often unknown, people, and the risk is increased or diminished according to their competence. This is what happens whenever we board a train and trust that the driver, signalman, linesmen and engineers know their jobs, or eat in a restaurant and trust in the staff that we will not get food poisoning. In other situations we are largely dependant on ourselves and the relative safety of the process derives from our own good sense, previous planning, and behaviour at the time. Going on a camping expedition or canoeing or sailing are situations of this kind. There may be variations in the natural order, changes in the weather, for example, which we must take into account, and it would be foolish to ignore such changes, but decisions are in our own hands and we make choices about what, how, and when we do things. Having a baby in hospital is a bit like getting on a plane and trusting the pilot. Having a baby at home is like going out in a sailing boat of which you are the captain.

Just as situations may occur in which the captain decides that the best thing is to make for the nearest harbour, so there are situations which can crop up in pregnancy or during labour which indicate that it is best to go to hospital. This is why it is vital for a woman to get full information about the progress of the pregnancy and labour and her and the baby's state so that she can make decisions of such a kind on the basis of knowledge. No woman should decide that she is going to have her baby at home whatever happens. It is important to maintain flexibility and to keep the option of hospital open should it be needed, and impossible to know for sure in advance. Enthusiasm for home birth should not blind us to the real advantages of hospital if there are clear indications of pathology. Birth at home is for normal deliveries following on straightforward pregnancies. There is then only a very slight risk of losing a baby; in England and Wales in 1970 only 4 out of every 1000 babies born at home died, and they would probably have died wherever they were born. The overall perinatal mortality figure, for births both in hospital and at home, was nearly 17 per 1000.

These figures are misleading in a way because stillbirths and neonatal deaths occurring in babies born of women who were moved to hospital during labour because of difficulties are recorded as hospital deaths, and this means that the perinatal mortality rate for home births is artificially lower than it should be. Even so, the risk of a baby dying is clearly very low indeed. What each woman has to decide is whether that is an acceptable risk to take.

Risk factors known before pregnancy

Although it is probably wrong to make hard and fast rules, because much depends on the strength of the woman's wish for birth at home, her health and social conditions, and on the skills of those available to help her, there are certain factors which suggest that there is a greater chance than usual of things not going in a straightforward way or of everything going well. Many of these can be known even before a pregnancy starts. They are discussed under four headings below.

The relation between parity, social class, age, and height

Parity describes the number of babies which a woman has previously had. From the obstetrician's point of view the woman having her first baby is an unknown quantity and therefore something of an obstetric risk. The one who has had four previous babies may also be at risk. In between the first and fourth births the chances of anything going wrong are low. It is possible to do all sorts of arithmetic to show that first births are slightly riskier than second ones. But by itself parity is not a very useful measurement. It must be taken in relation to age, the normality or otherwise of any previous pregnancies and labours, and (something which makes adverse comment on the society in which we live) social class. Wives of manual workers and unsupported mothers (including unmarried women and those who are divorced, separated or widowed) are in the highest-risk categories.

Although some statistics indicate that teenage pregnancies are higher risk than those in which the mother is older, this is not true for middle-class mothers. In fact, perinatal mortality (still births and deaths in the first week of life) is lowest of all in this group.

Mothers having their fifth babies whose four previous pregnancies and labours were normal and who are under 40 are also very likely to have a straightforward labour.

Birth at home

In fact, the middle- and upper-class mother has a much better chance of experiencing a normal pregnancy and labour and of giving birth to a live, healthy baby than the mother at the bottom of the social scale. At present the perinatal mortality of those in social class 5 is twice that of those in social class 1 (see Table 1).

TABLE 1: *Outcomes of births in different social classes**

Social class	Perinatal mortality rates
1	7.5
2	15.8
3	19.6
4	26.5
5	27.6
Unsupported mothers	37.4

*Adapted from W. M. O. Moore: Antenatal care and the choice of place of birth. In *The place of birth* (eds. Sheila Kitzinger and John Davis). Oxford University Press (1978).

Mothers in lower socio-economic classes are less likely to be healthy themselves, do not have such good diets, are more likely to smoke during pregnancy, tend to be less well built, are more likely to develop toxaemia in pregnancy, and their mothers, in their turn, tended to suffer these socio-economic disadvantages.

Physiologically the best age to have a first baby is before one is 30. Women having their first babies when they are 30 or more are called 'elderly' primigravidae. When a woman is feeling very happy about being pregnant and is healthy and full of vitality it is off-putting to hear this description. It does not mean that labour is likely to be difficult in her case, only that if one looks at the whole category of primigravidae of this age there will be comparatively more women who encounter difficulties.

Height has been shown to be another important variable. The shorter the mother, the more risk to her baby, the taller, the less the risk. But this is also associated with social class, women in higher social classes having usually had the kind of diet and social conditions in childhood which allowed them to grow to their optimum heights. Hospitals usually decide that a woman is short if she is less than 1.52 metres (5 feet) tall. If a short woman has a straightforward pregnancy and the baby's head engages in the pelvis shortly before the birth is due there is no reason why she should not have her baby at home.

Some women are genetically small-boned and short. A Chinese or Indian mother, for example, may be perfectly fit and yet come into the category of 'short', and she also tends to bear a smallish baby who may be considered to be of low birth weight (under 2.5 kg or 5.5 lb) although it has been well nourished in the uterus and is mature.

The weight of the previous baby

If the previous baby was of a good weight, the next one is also likely to grow well in the uterus and to be born at the right time. But if the last baby was of low birth weight the same factors may be present to produce a baby who is less well adapted to starting life and who may need special care. (Obviously this does not apply if the last birth produced twins.) Babies weighing 2.5 kilograms or less account for two-thirds of all perinatal deaths. It is the greatest single cause of perinatal mortality.[1] Most of these are premature babies, but probably as many as one-third of these low-weight babies are born at the right time but have not grown well in the uterus. If the previous baby was 2.5 kilograms or under the right place for delivery is a hospital with a *special-care baby-unit,* not home. For the same reason if a woman hopes for a home birth but goes into labour 3 weeks or more before her expected date there is a strong case to be made for going to hospital for the delivery, in case the baby needs special care.

The kind of labour a woman had previously

The woman who has had a difficult labour may have the same kind of labour again. On the other hand, if her previous labour took place in hospital there may have been factors related to hospital-style childbirth and obstetric intervention, for example, induction or acceleration or pain-relieving drugs, which in themselves have contributed to or even caused the complicated labour. Epidural anaesthesia greatly increases the chance of a woman needing a forceps delivery. For example, in one study women who had had elective epidurals had a five-times-greater

[1] W. M. O. Moore in *The place of birth,* op. cit.

chance of a forceps delivery.[1] So one should not automatically assume that a previous forceps delivery necessitates a hospital birth next time.

If a previous labour went well this is a good indication that the next labour is likely to go well or, since second labours are usually easier and quicker, even better.

Previous difficulties with the third stage

Postpartum haemorrhage and the need for manual removal of the placenta under anesthesia following a previous birth suggests that the same problem may crop up after another delivery. It is usually unwise to plan a home birth if this occurred. There is some evidence, however, that retention of the placenta, and the need for its manual removal, is more common when oxytocin has been used to induce labour. A woman who has had a previous labour with induction and other kinds of obstetric intervention the necessity for which is in question, might ask herself whether going to the same hospital and having high-technology care is more likely to produce the same third-stage abnormalities than staying at home and having her baby as naturally as possible. But if she decides on a home birth it is essential that she is within 20 minutes of the obstetric flying squad.

An antenatal prediction score has been outlined by the authors of the British Births 1970 Survey[2] which includes biological and social factors. They recommend that anyone scoring 4 or more should be delivered in hospital.

Second thoughts about home birth: difficulties that may arise during pregnancy

Toxaemia

Toxaemia (the short term for 'pre-eclamptic toxaemia'), the first sign of which is a rise in diastolic blood-pressure to 90 or more, may reduce the growth of the baby in the uterus. One in every four

[1] I. J. Hoult, A. H. MacLennan, and L. E. S. Carrie: Lumbar epidural anaesthesia in labour: relation to foetal malposition and instrumental delivery'. *British Medical Journal* i, 14 – 16 (1977).

[2] G. Chamberlain, E. Philipp, B. Howlett, and K. Masters: *British births 1970*, Vol. II *Obstetric care*. Heinemann, London (1978).

Safety

TABLE 2: *The antenatal prediction score*

Maternal age	Score
20 – 29	0
20 and 30 – 34	1
35 and over	2

Parity	
1 and 2	0
0 and 3	1
4 and over	2

Social class	
I and II	0
III	1
IV, V, and unemployed	2
Unsupported mothers (single, separated, divorced, and widows)	2

Previous obstetric performance*	
Stillbirth	4
Neonatal death	4
Abortion**	4
Caesarean section	4

Previous obstetric history	
Antepartum haemorrhage	2
Postpartum haemorrhage	4
Immature delivery 36 weeks or less	2
Low birthweight infant 2.5 kg or less	2

Previous or present medical history	
Cardiac disease	4
Chronic respiratory disease	4
Chronic renal disease	4
Endocrine disease	4
Hypertension (blood pressure 140/90 or more before 20 weeks gestation)	4
Diabetes	4
Height 62 inches	1
Smokes 5 cigarettes or more per day	1

*The obstetricians' choice of words, not mine.
**'Abortion' here means a spontaneous abortion, another term for miscarriage.

expectant mothers become hypertensive (the medical term for having high blood-pressure) at some stage of pregnancy. If toxaemia is allowed to become severe it may also lead to eclampsia, a condition in which the mother has fits, which puts her life at risk. This is why blood pressure is taken and tests done for the presence of protein in the urine during pregnancy.

Analysis of the 1970 births survey reveals that high blood-pressure by itself or linked with mild toxaemia is not associated with prematurity or with babies dying at or shortly after birth. Mild toxaemia and raised blood-pressure are in no way harmful. But the clinical evidence demonstrates that if the mother becomes *severely* pre-eclamptic (diastolic blood-pressure above 109) this can lead to delayed breathing or the baby may die. Even so, in 1970, 59 women with severe toxaemia had their babies at home and all the babies lived, 69 had their babies in GP units where the mortality rate was 29 per cent, and 669 gave birth in Consultant Units, where 33 babies (5 per cent) died. Although the authors of *British Births 1970* simply remark that 'it is probably fortuitous that no infant born to a severely pre-eclamptic mother at home died' and go on to recommend that all women with high blood-pressure should have their babies in Consultant Units, the data they present does not support their argument and in fact suggests that it is more dangerous to have a baby in a Consultant Unit than in one's own home!

If a woman becomes severely toxaemic her obstetrician may advise her to go into hospital for rest and sedation, and if foetal growth is slow or stops he or she will watch carefully until the right moment comes to induce labour. Since the baby may be immature and/or small-for-dates, labour should take place in a hospital where immediate paediatric care is available if needed.

Hypertension without other symptoms

Sometimes blood pressure goes up after about the 28th week of pregnancy only to go down again shortly afterwards. The mother may be able to stabilize her own blood pressure by rest, relaxation, and peace of mind. There is little scientific evidence to support the use of sedation and bedrest as a treatment for simple high blood-pressure when there is no albumin (protein) in the mother's urine and this is a poor reason for being admitted to hospital. A study[1] of women who were divided into

---

[1] D. D. Mathews: A randomized controlled trial of bedrest and sedation or normal activity and non-sedation in the management of non-albumineuric hypertension in late pregnancy. *British Journal of Obstetrics and Gynaecology* **84**, 108 – 14 (1977).

four treatment groups, one which had bedrest in hospital with sedatives, one with bedrest in hospital without sedatives, one with normal activity at home with sedatives, and one with normal activity at home without sedatives, revealed that babies in all four groups were of about the same weight and there were no significant differences in outcome between them. There is no reason why the woman with simple hypertension should not have a home birth.

The earlier that symptoms of toxaemia develop in pregnancy the less likely it is that the mother's health can be maintained in such a way that a home birth carries little risk.

Other problems

Anaemia is a contra-indication to home birth, since any blood loss could be dangerous for the mother. It is important that the haemoglobin level be checked and that if it is below 12.6 grams the mother must have iron and folic acid supplements. If in spite of this the haemoglobin (Hb on the record card) remains below this level, the birth should take place in hospital.

The baby who is presenting by the *breech* is safer being born in hospital because there is some chance of breathing difficulties. 10 out of every 100 breech babies are slow to breathe at delivery compared with only 2 babies born head-first. Many of these breech babies are also premature so special care should be available because of their immaturity.

Indications that *the baby is not growing well* in the uterus may also suggest that the birth should take place in hospital. But the woman who sees a different doctor at almost every antenatal visit need not worry about any remarks that may be made about the height of the fundus. This is the usual way in which uterine size is assessed, but an unreliable one, especially if different people see the mother at different visits. In an antenatal class of 16 women I learned that 5 having their babies in 4 London hospitals had had warnings about their babies being 'small'. All of them went on to deliver babies whose weights were well within the normal range. The rate of increase in the size of the uterus is more important than the height of the top of it in relation to the mother's umbilicus.

If *the mother has not felt the baby move for 10 hours* or if she is at all worried about the frequency and strength of foetal movements, she should see her doctor or go to the hospital and ask for an examination. When the foetus has engaged movements usually change in type and instead of the whole-body movements a woman experiences at about 28 – 38 weeks, only movements of thrusting head and hands, feet, elbows, and knees may be felt. Even these can sometimes be extraordinarily sharp. But when the baby is deep in the pelvis it cannot so easily move its whole body in the porpoise-like leaps and swoops of the earlier weeks. The vigorous baby continues to move limbs, however, at times when it is not sleeping. Any change in the nature of foetal movements is worth noting and reporting to the doctor. This is something the woman can do for herself. The baby who is not well stops moving and the birth should obviously take place in hospital where intensive care of the baby is possible after birth.

Vaginal bleeding after the first 3 – 4 months of pregnancy should always be reported to the doctor. This may be spotting from the cervix as it starts to efface and dilate in late pregnancy, a frequent occurrence. Sometimes, however, it is a symptom of the placenta lying beside or in front of the baby's head, *placenta praevia*. When there is suspected placenta praevia delivery must take place in hospital. Diagnosis can be made by ultrasound, but a scan in *early* pregnancy sometimes shows a low-lying placenta which proves later not to be the case.

If you go *more than two weeks 'overdue'* and are sure of your dates plans for a home birth may need to be changed. About 32 women in every 100 go past the expected date of delivery. Most women get anxious when they come up to the date and nothing happens. Doctors also become concerned when a woman goes past her dates because of the statistical association between postmaturity (42 weeks or more from the first day of the last menstrual period) and perinatal mortality, remarked on in various surveys. The British Births Survey of 1970,[1] however, revealed that labour is likely to be straightforward; in fact mothers who are 'overdue' have fewer operative deliveries than others. It also emerged that only 8 per 1000 babies died in weeks 41 and 42 and 18 in week 43 and after, rates lower than the 23 per 1000 for the survey as a whole.

Passionate love-making leading to orgasm can sometimes start off labour when the time is ripe. Alcohol inhibits uterine action to some extent so plenty of sex and no drinking can be a good prescription for initiating labour naturally.

[1] G. Chamberlain *et al.,* op. cit.

Safety

How to know that all is well

Go to the antenatal clinic regularly so that blood pressure, urine, etc. can be checked. Discuss the results with your doctor. Ask if you may have an explanation of notes on your record card. Screening for spina bifida and other neural-tube defects can be carried out by a blood test between the 16th and 18th weeks.

Get familiar with the way your baby moves, and notice when and where you feel the strongest movements. Note any marked variations from week to week.

Make sure that any bladder infection is promptly treated, since harmful bacteria can be one cause of renal infection in pregnancy and premature birth. A do-it-yourself kit can be bought from the chemist's to check the urine. Spend enough time on the lavatory to really empty the bladder, shifting position so that no urine is retained because of the position of the baby's head.

If abdominal girth is not measured in your antenatal clinic check the growth of the uterus yourself by passing a tape measure around your tummy at the level of the umbilicus every 2 weeks or so. It should measure an increasing amount, a sure sign that the baby is continuing to grow provided that you have no exceptional quantity of amniotic fluid.

Another sign of a straightforward labour is that the baby's head engages as term approaches (often several weeks before, but sometimes not until labour starts). When this happens the head goes deep into the pelvis like an egg in an egg-cup and the part of the baby which can be palpated abdominally is the trunk and buttocks, the head being down below the pubic bone. When this occurs the abdominal profile changes, which may be immediately obvious to your partner; you are 'slung lower'. If there were any difficulties in breathing, when for example you ran up stairs, these are now alleviated. On the other hand bladder frequency is common once the baby's head is pressing against the bladder and frequent, rather loose bowel motions may indicate that the head is pressing also against the rectum. Movements of the baby's head against the pelvic floor muscles may produce a sensation like a mild electric shock in the vagina, a sure sign that the head is very low.

A woman whose baby does not engage when she is lying down on an examination couch may find that when she stands up the head descends into the pelvis.

Birth at home

A woman having a baby at home should plan to have with her a skilled and experienced birth attendant, preferably one who is accustomed to doing home births. This is getting more and more difficult in Britain today because fewer GPs and midwives are doing home births, so that skills are being forgotten or never acquired. This constitutes an understandable reason for a doctor being reluctant to agree to do a home birth. One of the ways in which this problem may be circumvented is by finding out that hospital back-up would be available if necessary and that, should either the midwife or the GP need further assistance, they can contact one of the hospital obstetricians who is willing to come to the home. Some obstetric registrars are willing to do this if arrangements are made in advance. This can often be done through the senior community midwife in the area, and she is likely to know which obstetricians may be interested. A reluctant GP may feel much happier when he or she knows that this back-up is available, or may prefer to hand over to the midwife, who then calls in the hospital doctor if necessary.

A vital element in safety is good antenatal care. The woman planning home birth should have regular check-ups from the time she has missed her second period, if not before, and in the final weeks should have a weekly antenatal visit. Her blood pressure, urine, weight, and probably her abdominal girth, too, should be recorded and the foetal heart auscultated and the uterus palpated to determine the baby's lie and presentation and whether or not it has engaged, and she should have an opportunity to discuss foetal movements and also to talk about any problems and worries.

Emergencies during and following labour

Obstetric textbooks set out a long list of things that go wrong during and after labour, but although doctors and midwives need to understand these, going into labour burdened by a sense of possible pathology can do the pregnant woman nothing but harm. If a sailor spent his time reading about shipwrecks and disasters he might never summon up the courage to go to sea.

Good health, common sense, a calm mind, and careful, observant birth attendants go a long way toward avoiding complications. They cannot rule them out entirely. There remain three kinds of emergency which occasionally happen without prior warning, all of which are far less common at home than in hospital, and which are very unlikely to occur after a normal pregnancy, labour, and delivery but of which the woman should be aware. They are prolapse of the cord, the baby not breathing at delivery, and heavy bleeding in the mother.

Allowing gravity to help descent of the baby's head by keeping out of bed and moving around can almost always avoid prolapse of the umbilical cord, which occurs when the baby's head or other presenting part does not fit the cervix so that there is space for a loop of cord to slip down in front of it. When this happens the cord comes down and hangs from the vagina like a loop of hosepipe which is gelatinous and spiralled with blue and white like a barber's pole. The baby must then be delivered rapidly by Caesarean section. Sometimes blood can be kept pulsating through the cord for a short time by getting the mother on all fours with her bottom in the air and her head and forearms low. She should be got to hospital immediately and somone should telephone meanwhile to warn the hospital of the situation. This emergency is very unlikely to occur if the head has engaged before or as labour starts, but there is an incidence of about 1 in every 2000 births in apparently normal labours. This 1 might be prevented by upright posture and greater mobility in early labour.

The baby who does not breathe following delivery has always suffered distress during the labour. It never happens out of the blue. The foetal heart-rate should be checked regularly throughout labour so that the baby's condition is known. Unless delivery is imminent the mother whose baby is indicating distress should be moved to hospital. Some babies need help to take their first breaths. This is a matter of clearing the airways, which may be blocked with mucus, and the simplest way of doing this is by lying or holding the baby on its tummy so that its head is slighly lower than its buttocks and the mucus drains out by gravity. The baby splutters and sneezes so that it assists in clearing its own airways.

In hospital nearly all babies are routinely suctioned with a suction nozzle passed into the mouth 'just in case'. Some people consider it an unnecessary assault on a baby who is already peacefully breathing and that it is another example of interventionist techniques which have come to be accepted as part of normal practice. Even those who deliver at home sometimes think it is important to have mucous catheters available, and this is one of the objects on the list recommended by the Association for Childbirth at Home to prepare for a home birth. This is not only unnecessary but could even be harmful. Dr Donald Garrow says, 'Sticking a catheter down a baby's throat is bad. Pushing it into a baby's mouth and nose does nothing at all to help it breathe. Mucus catheters should be banned as dangerous instruments'.[1]

The old idea that babies need smacking on the bottom is incorrect. A baby who has had a traumatic delivery does not need yet another shock. Most babies who are drowsy and slow to breathe at delivery have received high doses of analgesic or anaesthetic drugs from their mothers' blood stream, and it is rare for a newborn to have breathing difficulties if it is not drugged. Respiratory depression is unlikely to happen at home because drugs in such high doses are not given.

Babies whose mothers have received pethidine (or pethilorfan) within 4 – 5 hours or delivery may need some stimulation to breathe because they have not had time to eliminate the drug and are doped.[2] Analgesic drugs should be kept to the minimum in home births.

While the cord is still pulsating the baby is getting its oxygen supply from the mother's blood stream and there is no need to do anything about its breathing. The cord usually throbs for about 2 minutes and while it continues to do so it should not be clamped or cut until the baby is breathing well. Keeping the baby below the level of the placenta (which is still inside the uterus) until the cord has stopped pulsating allows all available oxygen and blood to be conveyed to the newborn, so until the baby is breathing independently it is probably best kept lying over the mother's thigh.

Five times more babies have difficulty in breathing in hospital than at home.[3] This suggests either that there is good selection of women for home birth or that procedures common in hospital, such as induction and acceleration of labour, and the use of narcotic drugs and anaesthesia, produce respiratory depression in some babies.[4] It is probably a combination of these factors which results in home-delivered babies breathing more easily.

[1] Personal communication

[2] M. I. J. Hogg, P. C. Wiener, M. Rosen, and W. W. Mapleson: Urinary excretion of pethidene and norpethidene in the newborn. *British Journal of Anaesthesia* **49** (9), 891 – 9 (1977).

[3] G. Chamberlain *et al., op. cit.*

[4] W. M. O. Moore, In *The Place of Birth, op. cit.*

Safety

The term 'respiratory depression' is used when a baby takes more than 3 minutes before taking its first breath. Some midwives now carry apparatus to resuscitate a baby who is slow to breathe, in the form of a Penlon bag.[1] It should not be used if meconium, the first bowel movements, is present in the amniotic fluid lest the baby may have inhaled it and it is forced into the lungs. This apparatus enables the airways to be cleared and also has a face-mask through which the baby can be given oxygen. A safety device is incorporated so that the lungs cannot be over-inflated. Ventilation rates of 60 per minute can be achieved. Other cheaper, disposable models are also on the market.

A light-weight mini-oxygen-cylinder which contains 20 minutes' supply of oxygen is also available and can be used either for the mother or the baby. It is refilled after use by the laboratory.

Another, more drastic way of getting a baby to breathe, is to intubate down between the vocal chords and give oxygen. Intubation should only be done by a paediatrician who has experience in this very difficult procedure. It means that the baby likely to have breathing problems should always be born in hospital and that there should be a paediatrician present at delivery. If a baby does not breathe and enormous effort is required to resuscitate it I believe that it is better stillborn than to survive brain-damaged. But it is important that parents deciding on birth at home think through this rare possibility in advance and discuss their own beliefs.

The third emergency occurs when in the third stage of labour the placenta starts to separate but fails to do so completely, so that there is bleeding from the sinuses in which the 'roots' of the placenta have been situated. Once the uterus can contract strongly these will be closed automatically. The treatment is to get the uterus to contract. This is why the midwife carries Syntocin which is usually given by injection as the baby is delivered. An alternative method of causing uterine contractions is to put the baby to the breast; the baby who is stimulating the nipple creates contractions. If the baby is not ready to suckle, the nipple can be stimulated by hand. The mother can also encourage her uterus to contract by gently massaging it with her hand. She will not cause herself pain, so it is safer for her to do this than for an inexperienced person to

[1] Longworth Scientific Instrument Co. Ltd—Cost about £30 at the time of writing.

41

do so. So long as there is only a little bleeding there is no danger in a prolonged third stage of one to two hours. The rapid third stages of 5 or 10 minutes often expected in hospital deliveries are not necessary at home and are a product of hospital organization. But someone should always watch for blood loss. The normal blood loss following delivery is about half a pint. Since the blood is mixed with amniotic fluid this cannot be gauged very accurately, but a bowl or kidney dish should be put to receive the blood so that it can be measured approximately.

If there is heavy bleeding and the placenta is not delivered, medical aid must be sought. It may be that a blood transfusion (the maternal blood-group should always be known in advance) and manual removal of the placenta are necessary. This is done under anaesthesia and is best performed in the home; ideally the mother should not be moved. In Britain obstetric 'flying squads' exist for such emergencies. Unfortunately in some areas these have been disbanded, a retrogessive step which resulted recently in a completely unnecessary maternal death. It is worth checking through your GP or the Community Health Council that the flying squad operates in your area; it should be able to reach you within half an hour of being summoned. It is the responsibility of consultants in each National Health Service region to maintain the flying squad in working order. In the absence of a flying squad in the area, you should be nearer still to the hospital.

Clearly, unless all births take place in an optimum environment some emergencies will occur and occasionally a baby will die. But at the present stage of knowledge, we do not know exactly what that environment is. A setting which is optimal for one woman and for one kind of labour may not be optimal for another woman and a labour of a different kind. There is no doubt that complicated labours should take place in hospital, and babies who are 'at risk' should be born there, but we cannot infer from this that all labours should take place in hospital and that straightforward labours and normal, healthy babies do best in a hospital setting.

The concept of an optimal environment for birth is useful only if it is related to specific circumstances and particular people. What is right for one mother and one baby may be quite wrong for another. Because it is a good thing for some children to have tonsillectomies we cannot conclude that all children should have their tonsils out, although this is more or less what happened 30 years ago when the fashion for tonsillectomies was at its height. The important thing is correct diagnosis so that tonsils are not removed when they are better left in. Moreover if people who do not really need operations have them none the less, they are exposed to risks to which they would not otherwise be subjected. When tonsillectomies were done most frequently some children suffered from the bad effects of anaesthesia and a few even died who would not otherwise have done so.

When intensive medical or obstetric care is extended to all sections of the population regardless of their individual requirements it is almost invariably spread thin. When special-care baby-units are filled with babies who do not need care of this kind, the babies who do are likely to get less careful attention than if only those babies who really need the observation and treatment there go to special care.

Similarly, if every woman in labour is in intensive care in a high-technology hospital, surrounded by sophisticated equipment, and attended by doctors who are experts in dealing with pathological conditions, the women who really benefit from this kind of care tend to get less concentrated attention.

Moreover if high-technology obstetrics in a hospital environment is the only kind of maternity care available, doctors and midwives do not get the training or practical experience in natural birth.

Midwives and women doctors tend to be the most anxious expectant mothers. They have seen all the things that can go wrong and approach childbirth with pathology dominant in their minds. This very anxiety may contribute to certain pathological conditions, such as uterine inertia (when the uterus fails to contract effectively) in which the anxious mind can affect the body.

Midwives often get little opportunity to see truly normal childbirth nowadays. They learn about pathology and drugs, sonar scans, monitors, and active management, but in many hospitals they know less and less about giving emotional support to their patients, how to help them through stressful phases in labour without recourse to the hypodermic syringe or the epidural. There is so much for the student midwife to learn about modern technology that there seems to be little time to cover these apparently less important aspects of midwifery, certainly ones which find a less obvious place in examination papers.

Student midwives in many areas get no chance to go out onto the district and do home deliveries; this is a deterioration in their training. Those who do see natural birth occurring under optimal conditions in the home or a friendly GP unit are often surprised that birth can be like this. A midwifery tutor remarked that her students were often startled by the mother's ease and happiness and by the whole atmosphere of this kind of birth when they had come from the first six months of their training in the Consultant Unit.

There is evidence that once a certain proportion of hospital births (which probably varies with different communities) is attained the perinatal mortality rate does not drop further even though all mothers are admitted to hospital to have their babies. This was observed in Cardiff where an intensive study of the effects of maternity care was conducted over an 8-year period during which women were not allowed to have their babies at home. In fact Cardiff perinatal mortality rates did not go down during all those years—a time during which a sophisticated technology had been introduced in the hospitals and when perinatal mortality rates in other parts of the British Isles were reduced.[1] It has been suggested that about 40 per cent of births could take place at home with relative safety if this is what women want, and that increasing hospital births beyond approximately 60 per cent does not add to safety.[2]

Since we do not understand all the factors which make for optimal care in different kinds of labours, it may also be that to take women into hospital who do not need it and to bring up the full range of diagnostic and other technical apparatus to 'actively manage' their labours may actually make the environment worse for them than if they had been in their own homes. Certainly this is what some women who have had distressing labours believe. They feel that if they had been allowed to labour in their own way, at their own pace, in an environment in which they felt at ease, labour might have been very different for them.

This is where antenatal care and correct diagnosis on the basis of which advice can be given to women of where the birth should take place is vitally important. Obstetricians see it in terms of good 'selection' of patients. I prefer to see it in terms of choices the woman is given together with information and guidance on which

[1] I. Chalmers, J. E. Zlosnik, K. A. Johns, and H. Campbell: Obstetric practice and outcome of pregnancy in Cardiff residents, 1965-1973. *British Medical Journal* **i,** 735 (1976).
[2] Martin Richards In *The Place of Birth,* op. cit.

she can come to her own decision. Sometimes the doctor may not agree with her. If the obstetrician believes she is wrong she should be urged to seek another opinion which she can weigh against the first. But in the end it *is* she who must decide.

Comparative statistics on perinatal mortality

Comparisons between countries in which most births take place at home or in hospital suggest that the place where birth occurs is less important than the social conditions in which the parents live. The West European country with the largest number of doctors per head of the population, Italy, also has a high perinatal mortality rate. The relative safety or danger of childbirth reflects wealth and poverty, education and ignorance, and the other social divisions which separate the haves from the have-nots. This is shown clearly in the international statistics for perinatal mortality in Table 3.

TABLE 3: *Perinatal mortality*
(includes stillbirths and deaths within the first week of life)*

	Perinatal mortality per 1000 births		
	1969	*1973*	*Most recent*
United States	27.1		20.5 (1975)
England and Wales	23.7	21.3	17.0 (1977)
Scotland	25.6	22.7	18.3 (1977)
Northern Ireland	29.2	25.9	25.9 (1975)
Republic of Ireland	27.0		22.0 (1974)
Sweden	16.3	12.9 (1974)	10.7 (1976)
Norway	20.7	16.8	13.3 (1976)
Finland	18.9		13.9 (1974)
Netherlands	19.6	16.4	13.9 (1975)
Belgium	25.1		19.5 (1975)
France	25.4		19.3 (1974)
Italy	32.4		23.8 (1975)
West Germany	25.2	23.2	19.3 (1975)
Switzerland	19.5	15.5	13.1 (1976)

*Data made available by the Department of Health and Social Security.

Birth at home

The figures must be treated with caution because the assessment of stillbirth varies between countries, some reckoning a stillbirth one which others term as abortion. In France and Italy, for example, the perinatal mortality figures count stillbirths from 26 weeks, and in the U.S.A. from as early as 20 weeks. The corrected 1975 rate for the U.S.A. (i.e. from 28 weeks) is 17.7—quite a difference!

Sweden has the lowest perinatal mortality rate in the world. 1.5 brain-damaged babies per 1000 are sent to special institutions, compared with 5.4 per 1000 in the U.S.A. Nearly every baby is born in hospital and it is tempting to explain the safety of birth in Sweden by its 100-per-cent hospital-delivery rate. But we cannot make any *causal* inference from the figures. The Netherlands also has a very low perinatal mortality rate and the same proportion of brain-damaged babies; yet about half its babies are born at home.

The Dutch home-birth system

The trend in Holland is towards more and more hospital births and there is a 2 per cent per annum decline in home births, since obstetricians who have done postgraduate training in the USA, Britain, or elsewhere are impressed by the new technology of childbirth in those countries, and believe that if this is used they may be able to save more babies.

This movement towards hospital births is also a struggle over who has control of childbirth—obstetricians or midwives. The first midwifery schools in the Netherlands were started in 1865. Traditionally midwives who are very highly trained, with a 3-year midwifery education, compared with a 2-year one in the United Kingdom, for example, have been the only attendants at normal childbirth, and it is they who have decided when and if it is necessary to call in a doctor and whether to move the mother to hospital if things are not going well. Domiciliary midwives have professional status, their own consulting rooms which mothers visit to have their pregnancies confirmed and for antenatal care, maintain a one-to-one relationship with their patients throughout the pregnancy, labour, and the postpartum period, and are able to care for 100 − 200 women a year. They can do this because they also have their own attendants, trained maternity-aid nurses (*kraamverzorgsters*) who care for the mother and family, being on duty from 7 a.m. till the husband returns in the evening, and forming an important part of the home care team. Professor

Safety

Kloosterman, Professor of Obstetrics at the University of Amsterdam, a great believer in home births and a champion of the rights of midwives, writes that the function of the doctor/nurse team in the hospital is to deal with pathology. The home care team is meant to 'protect a healthy woman during pregnancy and childbirth and to give her careful observation and mental support.'[1]

Maternity-aid nurse training in Holland first started in 1904. It is a 15-month course which includes hygiene, the care of mother and new-born baby, cookery, budgeting for meals, and looking after toddlers. It is much sought in the Netherlands; the image of the young nurse who is capable enough to run a home, look after a woman, help establish breastfeeding, care for a toddler, and cook an evening meal for the family before she leaves when the husband comes home from work, is an attractive one to the Dutch. The turnover in maternity-aid nurses is rapid, because the marriage rate is high. No similar training exists anywhere else in the world. But it is an important part of the home-birth system in the Netherlands and one without which the midwife would be occupied with simple nursing tasks instead of concentrating on midwifery.

When there are no indications that hospital birth is necessary the Dutch health-insurance scheme pays the midwife's fee and most of the costs of the maternity-aid nurse.

In the Netherlands women, instead of being 'selected' for home birth, as in Britain, are selected for hospital birth. If there are any indications of abnormality the woman knows that she must go to hospital. These include toxaemia, hypertension, and signs of disproportion between the baby and the maternal pelvis. A woman having her first baby automatically goes to hospital if she is aged 35 or more, one having her second or subsequent baby if she is 45 or more. If labour is premature or does not start until after 42 weeks she also goes to hospital. Social conditions are also taken into account: there should be adequate heating in the home, a lavatory on the same floor, and the means to get the woman to hospital within an hour if necessary.

Obstetricians often shake their heads over the Dutch system and its associated low perinatal mortality rate. Many question the validity of some of the Dutch statistics, especially those concerning death from birth trauma, which are remarkably low in Holland, and assert that if all babies were born in hospital the rate could be

[1] In *The place of birth,* op. cit.

even lower. The perinatal mortality rate for home births *including* those transferred to hospital during labour and delivered in hospital (in contrast to the way in which the figures are arrived at for England and Wales), is 4.5 per 1000, and for all births 16 per 1000. Opponents of home birth explain this by saying that it is because Holland is such a small country and the roads are so good that women can get to hospital quickly and doctors to them. Although this is undoubtedly one factor in a safe system it is doubtful that it can completely account for the figures. They also suggest that the Dutch women are all well built and have ample pelvises. Yet the Dutch population includes a large proportion of immigrants from Indonesia, the West Indies, and the Mediterranean area, countries in which the perinatal mortality rate is much higher. Another argument is that it must be the dairy products or because Dutch women are 'sensible' and homely. One gets the impression that there must be a stereotype of Dutch women as flaxen-haired apple-cheeked Nordic mother-figures, with ample bosoms, wide hips, and placid minds, busy with home tasks, contented with their lot, and perhaps wearing those delightful lace and linen headdresses which are donned by models working for the Cheese Board to advertize Gouda and Edam. Television coverage associated with Moluccan protest and terrorism should have corrected this picture, but such is the force of national stereotypes that it may not have done so.

Professor Kloosterman believes that the home-birth system in the Netherlands has built-in advantages and says that:

In her own home the expectant mother is not considered a patient, but a woman fulfilling a natural and highly personal task. She is the real centre around which everything (and everybody) revolves. The midwife or doctor and the maternity-aid nurse are all her guests, there to assist her. This setting reinforces her self-respect and self-confidence. The modern hospital very often functions in an opposite way. The woman is the guest of the doctors and nurses in *their* home. She becomes a patient, dependant on people who like to mother her. The security of the hospital, so important in situations where interference is necessary, is of no use for women who do not need any interference. The atmosphere in the hospital on the other hand weakens her self-confidence. This explains why in many hospitals (and in many countries with total hospitalization) the percentage of artificial deliveries is rising to such an extent that it is inconceivable that it occurs for good medical reasons.[1]

[1] *The place of birth,* op. cit.

Safety

The rate of perinatal mortality in Holland has been falling along with the rates in most other countries where social conditions have improved over the last 50 years. In Holland the perinatal mortality rate for births at home has also fallen dramatically over the same period. It was 14 per 1000 in 1960 and as we have seen was down to just over 4 per 1000 by 1974, a figure which (although not directly comparable because of different statistical practices) is the same as that for home births in England and Wales. The perinatal mortality rate for hospital births in Holland in the same year was 23 per 1000 (we do not know the rate for England and Wales as deaths and births were not linked statistically in terms of where they occurred until 1975). This does not mean that home was safer than hospital, but that those women who needed to go to hospital had hospital deliveries.

Other countries

In assessing the meaning of perinatal mortality statistics in different countries demographic factors are very important.

Even if medical practice had remained unchanged in Europe and North America, maternal and perinatal mortality would have continued to fall because of the relatively greater decline in fertility rates among groups at increased risk of maternal and perinatal death . . . 27 per cent of the improvement in the United States infant mortality rate between 1965 and 1970 and at least one-third of the observed improvement in the England and Wales maternal mortality rate between 1964–66 and 1970–72 was due to secular changes in maternal age and parity.[1]

What this means is that women who do not want babies, who are unfit for childbearing, or who are likely to bear particularly high-risk babies for genetic or other reasons, because of contraception and more readily available legal termination of pregnancy need no longer have babies; that smaller families tend to result in mothers who are in better health who are not worn out by childbearing and rearing; that women finish childbearing at an earlier age and so are not exposed to the extra risks of having babies at around the time of the menopause (although this is partially offset by the fact that women are also starting their families later); and that improved social and economic conditions further cut down the risks of

---

[1] I. Chalmers and M. Richards: in *Benefits and hazards of the new obstetrics* (ed. Tim Chard and Martin Richards). Heinemann, London (1977).

childbirth. To attribute the reduction in perinatal mortality to improvements in medical care or obstetric skills confuses association with cause and effect. In a study of home and hospital births in Newcastle upon Tyne between 1960 and 1969 it was discovered that perinatal mortality dropped uniformly in both categories, although death rates still remained higher in hospital than in home deliveries.[1]

Once the perinatal mortality figures are down to 4.5 per 1000 (as they are with home births in Britain and Holland) there is unlikely to be any further marked improvement until there is the ability to control the development of the baby in the uterus in such a way that developmental abnormalities and genetic mishaps can be eradicated. Abnormalities of this kind exist in about the same proportion of births in England and Wales as in Holland and Sweden. Congenital malformations accounted for 2 deaths in the first month of life out of every 1000 babies born alive in England and Wales, the Netherlands, and Sweden in 1973.

Hospital perinatal mortality rates could be further reduced if pre-term births could be avoided (since most premature births take place in hospital, as they should) and if placental function could be improved so that there were no underweight babies. There was a surprising rise in the perinatal mortality rate of England and Wales in the late sixties which was almost entirely due to the number of low-birth-weight babies who were born in that year (when induction of labour was at the height of its popularity). Sweden and the other Scandinavian countries have a very low proportion of low-birth-weight babies. This is associated with generally good nutrition and healthy mothers and little socio-economic differentiation between different occupational and other sections of society.

Ever since the nineteenth century such social changes have had the major impact on patterns of health and disease in the West, and the contribution made by medicine has followed on and complemented initiatives taken by lay people to create conditions for healthier living. 'The sanitary revolution that started in England in the 1830s . . . is responsible for modern water supplies and sewage, government departments of health and sanitary laws

[1] S. L. Barron, A. M. Thomson, and P. R. Philips: Home and hospital confinement in Newcastle upon Tyne, 1960 – 1969. *British Journal of Obstetrics and Gynaecology* **84**, 6 (1977).

50

and . . . our entire attitude towards cleanliness and health.'[1] It has done more to prevent disease than any miracle drug or surgery.

The place where a baby is born is less important than these large-scale socio-economic changes and resulting improvement in the health of whole populations. It is this which goes a long way toward explaining the extremely low perinatal mortality in countries like Sweden and Norway where poverty has been virtually eliminated. The most dramatic changes have occurred in Japan, where socio-economic factors have played a major part in reducing perinatal mortality by half between 1952 and 1972[2] (see Tables 4 and 5). It is not exclusively or predominantly new obstetric

TABLE 4: *Foetal, neonatal, and post-natal mortality per 1000 live births in selected countries, 1955 and 1973*

	Late foetal mortality (28 wks +)		% fall	Neonatal mortality (0 – 27 days)		% fall	Post-neonatal mortality (28 – 364 days)		% fall
	1955	1973		1955	1973		1955	1973	
Sweden	17.0	7.2	57.6	12.9	7.8	39.5	4.5	2.0	55.6
Japan	30.8	12.2	60.4	22.3	7.4	66.8	17.4	3.9	77.6
Finland	18.2	7.1	61.0	18.6	8.5	54.3	11.1	2.1	81.1
France	17.5	12.1	30.9	20.8	8.5	59.1	17.8	4.8	73.0
Netherlands	17.3	9.1	47.4	14.0	8.5	39.3	6.1	3.0	50.8
England and Wales	23.7	11.6	51.1	17.0	11.1	34.7	7.6	5.7	25.0

TABLE 5: *Gross national product* per capita

	Amount 1973 (U.S. $)	Growth rates (%) 1960 – 73	1965 – 73
Sweden	5910	3.0	2.4
France	4540	4.7	5.0
Netherlands	4330	4.1	4.3
Japan	3630	9.4	9.6
Finland	3600	4.5	5.2
United Kingdom	3060	2.4	2.3

[1] Eric J. Cassell: *The healer's art.* Penguin, Harmondsworth (1978).
[2] Eva Alberman in *Benefits and hazards of the new obstetrics,* op. cit.

techniques which are responsible for the drop in mortality but a rise in the standard of living.

So the challenge to prevent pre-term births and underweight babies is a matter for wider social changes, not one for the medical profession alone.

Yet even changed social conditions cannot entirely account for the drop in the perinatal mortality rate. West Germany has almost no home births and a standard of living which is higher than that of Holland, yet has a higher perinatal mortality rate (23 per 1000). The use of pain-relieving drugs in labour may make the journey to birth especially dangerous for some babies, and wide variations in the amount of analgesia used in different countries may introduce increased risk for the baby. In Britain 90 per cent of women have drugs for pain relief as compared with 20 per cent in Sweden and only 5 per cent in Holland. Woman tend to need more drugs when there is more obstetric intervention.

Professor Kloosterman believes that having a baby at home actually 'protects women against unnecessary interference' and that 'the presence of sophisticated equipment sometimes leads to it being used just because it is there. If you have to move a patient you have time to *think* whether it is necessary.'[1] It may be that this is one important factor in contributing towards the relative safety of having a baby at home. Another factor in making for safe childbirth is the skilled midwife. Finland has 100 per cent hospital-births and a low perinatal mortality rate. Midwives have high status and excellent training and most babies are delivered by them. The same is true for Sweden with its 100 per cent hospital-birth rate and for Holland with its home birth rate of nearly 50 per cent. In all those countries where obstetricians have taken over maternity care and the midwife has either virtually ceased to exist, as in the USA, or where her status and responsibility has been reduced to that of an assistant to the obstetrician, the perinatal mortality rates have not been reduced so rapidly as in those countries where the midwife has high status and personal responsibility for the conduct of labour.

It must be said, however, that the argument about home versus hospital birth can never be resolved at our present stage of

---

[1] Personal communication.

knowledge. Eva Alberman[1] says that 'a true comparison of home versus institutional delivery will never be achieved until it is possible to study outcomes such as the long-term quality of births in terms of physical, psychological, and mental health, the benefit to the mother of relief of pain or anxiety, the long-term benefit in terms of incidence of complications such as prolapse or urinary incontinence, and other similar measures.' The relative safety of home and hospital birth really includes all these different aspects of physical and psychological well-being. It is not just a matter of pushing out a live baby, a question of mere survival of mother and child, but of the quality of life which follows.

[1] *Benefits and hazards of the new obstetrics,* op. cit.

4

The baby born at home

BIRTH at home provides an environment in which not only a child, but a family, is born spontaneously. In my own study of mothers' reasons for choosing birth at home[1] about half of them stated as the main reason for their choice their concern that bonding with the baby should be able to take place naturally without interference by hospital staff and that there should be no separation from the newborn.

It is interesting that none of the women having their first babies mentioned this as the primary reason for wanting a home birth but every single one of the women who had already had babies in hospital wrote about it, often at length. One woman, for example, described how her baby had been brought to her in hospital:

. . . wrapped up in what looked like a little strait jacket, and I was ordered not to unwrap her to look at her or to try to change her, and to keep her on the outside of the bed-linen . . . . Like any mother, I longed to take off all her clothes and see how she looked, and hold her warm little body against my bare skin, but the nurse kept coming in or sat at the foot of the bed watching, so I didn't dare. . . . I had to convince myself that she really was my baby. When you've waited around for nine months to see your baby, it's very hard to be told you can see it only on schedule and it really won't be yours to take care of for a few more days.

Another said that she only had 'one glimpse of my red and sleepy little son who had been whisked away and put behind glass'.

Later the baby was brought to her:

I had an uncontrollable curiosity to find out about him—watch his funny little movements, take his clothes off and examine all his fingers and toes. I think this process of getting to know your baby in the physical sense is underestimated in the very beginning—that women do in fact need long periods of privacy when they can be allowed just to watch their baby and to

[1] Sheila Kitzinger and John Davis (Eds.): *The place of birth*. Oxford University Press (1978).

explore his or her body. I remember the feeling of never wanting to let him go from my bed. I wanted him to be with me, and I felt it a terrible deprivation when he was taken away to the nursery. I resented the fact that nurses were changing his nappy, picking him up, etc. when he was a part of me, and I couldn't wait to leave the hospital and have him to myself! . . . I longed to get home to total involvement with my baby.

Many women express a passionate sense of urgency about being able to care for their babies themselves from the first seconds of life and feel that only in the home environment can they be sure that this is possible. Although hospitals are now replacing the central nurseries which were designed on the American hospital model and are going back to having babies with their mothers for much of the time, we have seen that the design of wards, even the modern 4 – 6 bedded ones, means that babies are usually removed from their mothers at night to enable the women to sleep. It is a very different matter for a woman to wake and roll over, lift her baby from a cot at the bedside and cuddle it up to her breast, perhaps falling asleep while the baby is still sucking and waking to find it still nestled against her body. The disturbance is minimal and both mother and baby get the chance of extended flesh-to-flesh contact and loving closeness.

Many mothers instinctively feel that a crying newborn baby needs their immediate attention. In hospital, as we have seen, they lie awake wondering if the sounds of distress from the nursery are coming from *their* babies. A screaming baby alone in its cot or lined up with rows of other screaming newborns is a neglected baby. He cannot know that help is near, that milk is coming in half an hour or twenty minutes or even five minutes. He cannot know that loving arms are waiting to hold him. He is to all intents and purposes completely isolated and abandoned.

Some mothers also express anxiety about viral infections which can flare up in hospital nurseries. Echo II, a flu-like virus, infected 11 babies in a Cambridge special-care baby-unit over Christmas 1977 and three of them died. Cross-infection in nurseries means that epidemics can spread like wild-fire.

In both Consultant Units and GP units women are still sometimes separated from their babies who are cared for at least part of the 24 hours in communal nurseries. One woman wrote:

I think I encountered all that is worst in hospital care. The babies were kept in

The baby born at home

the nursery except for an exactly timed 30 minutes at each feed. There were constant injunctions 'not to touch that baby', 'put it down' and so on. Consequently I left hospital with a strange baby. I had no idea whether she cried between feeds always, sometimes or never. It took me at least six weeks to like her at all, which I feel can be attributed to the GP unit rules. It certainly left me feeling totally inadequate as a mother, and really unused to physical contact with my baby.

After a home birth women wrote vividly about the experience of meeting and getting to know their babies:

Later that night, when I was too happy to sleep, I took the baby from his cot and held him against my shoulder for the rest of the night. I seemed to breathe in his very essence and he I believe mine, too. I heard a psychologist once remark that a mother feels a sense of loss when her baby is born. I felt quite the opposite. Every part of me seemed to fill with what I can only describe as 'a loving ecstasy'. This intense communication (for I am sure it was two-way) was never possible in hospital immediately after birth as the babies were not beside me. But I wonder too if there it could have taken place. It was something so special I think it needed exactly the right receptive conditions on both our parts for it to happen.

The study of interaction between mothers and their young started with research on animals and birds. Human beings are not rats or birds, however. Although a deer or goat will not acknowledge her own young if she is anaesthetized at delivery and shown her offspring immediately after, common sense tells us that this is not so with human beings. We know, too, that human babies do not get imprinted by the first moving object they see like Lorenz's geese[1] or most of them would be attached to the midwives and doctors who delivered them. Yet recent research on human behaviour indicates that what happens in the minutes and hours following childbirth is important for human mothers and babies too. With nearly 100 percent hospital deliveries, the institutional organization of birth as if it were a surgical operation and resulting emphasis on asepsis, and the taking over of the baby by the hospital while the mother is nursed separately except for specific times when it is brought to her for feeding and for teaching her some of the manual crafts of mothering, interaction betweeen mother and baby is adversely affected in ways that have clear short-term and sometimes marked long-term consequences.

[1] Konrad Z. Lorenz: *King Solomon's Ring,* Methuen, London (1955).

Birth at home

In human beings most that is involved in parenting is not instinctive. It is *learned* behaviour, for both fathers and mothers.[1] When the environment does not facilitate that learning, a man or woman may become an inadequate parent unable to relate positively to the baby, and getting none of the satisfaction of the dialogue that can take place with a baby right from the beginning and continue, undergoing enormous changes on the way, into adulthood.

The newborn baby is well prepared for an environment in which interaction with its parents can start immediately after birth. It is an extraordinarily active, aware, sensitive, responsive creature, sending out signals to his or her caretakers if they only have eyes to see. It is not enough to pick up, put down, unwrap, clean, change, reclothe, and feed a baby. Human beings become fully human because they are treated like human beings.[2]

The work of Spitz,[3] Bowlby,[4] Winnicott,[5] and others shows how babies who are treated as if they are not human, who are handled like inanimate packages and who do not have one loving person to care for them, are slow to develop and tend to suffer many emotional and learning difficulties as they grow older.

Women need their babies with them if they are to grow into mothers, and babies need to be with their mothers if they are to start the conversation which has been called the synchronized 'dance',[6,7] which helps them grow into full human beings. All the transactions which are the basis of living in society start with this synchronized interaction of mother and baby.[8]

Aidan Macfarlane has drawn attention to the way in which hospital staff have often regarded babies as if they had no sensibilities. Yet in fact the sensitivity of a new born baby to harsh lights, loud, sudden noises, rough handling, heat and cold, and

[1] Sheila Kitzinger: *Women as mothers*. Fontana, London (1978).

[2] John and Elizabeth Newson: *Infant care in an urban community*. Allen & Unwin, London (1963).

[3] R. A. Spitz *et al.*: *The first year of life*. International Universities Press, New York (1965).

[4] John Bowlby: *Attachment and loss,* Vol. I, Penguin, Harmondsworth (1971).

[5] D. W. Winnicott: *Collected papers*. Tavistock (1958).

[6] Daniel Stern: *The first relationship: mother and child*. Fontana, London (1978).

[7] H. R. Schaffer: *Studies in mother – infant interaction*. Academic Press, London (1977).

[8] Sheila Kitzinger: *The experience of breastfeeding*. Penguin, Harmondsworth (1979).

The baby born at home

painful stimuli in general may be comparable with or greater than those of an adult: 'We still find it acceptable (though ever less so) to, by circumcision, remove a considerable area of extremely sensitive skin from the newborn without anaesthetic, and subject them, in special-care baby units, to procedures which an adult could never endure without the benefit of sedation or analgesia.'[1]

The Leboyer prose – poem[2] and film have focused on ways in which a baby can be welcomed into life with gentleness and love. Women have written to me of their distress in seeing their babies handled without tenderness and being treated as if they were hunks of meat.

Macfarlane describes how in one hospital (in a unit noted for its humanity) the average time for the baby to be with the mother after birth was 6.5 minutes, with a variation between 1 minute and 15 minutes.[3] This is very different from what happens at home, where everything that is done to or for the baby is done where the mother can see and share in the action, and where usually all this takes place right beside or actually on her bed. As mother and midwife start caring for the baby they do so as women participating together in the introduction of the baby to life and a common concern to make the newborn as comfortable as possible. They talk to each other and they both talk to the baby. This often does not occur in the hospital delivery room where a team approach to childbirth, rather than one-to-one relationships, creates a setting in which any conversation may be inhibited, where the person most in authority tends to address the mother exclusively by asking questions and giving instructions, and where the student midwife or junior hospital doctor often feels that the task in which he or she is engaged prohibits the time-wasting involved in having a conversation with a new-born baby. After the prescribed few minutes for officially sanctioned 'bonding', in many hospitals the baby is removed so that the team can proceed with delivery of the placenta, suturing of the mother's perineum, cleaning up, paediatric examination of the newborn, and all the other processes that must be completed before the mother can be moved to the postpartum ward and the delivery room prepared for the next patient.

In contrast, a mother who has her baby with her in the same room and who cares for him herself from the beginning can make of the beginnings of life a positive experience, full of loving touch and sounds, with which

[1] *The place of birth,* op. cit.
[2] Frédérick Leboyer: *Birth without violence.* Fontana, London (1977).
[3] *The place of birth,* op. cit.

the baby was already familiar in the uterus, and of her own voice.
John Kennell observed some profound differences between what
occurred after hospital deliveries and home births in California.[1]
This is how he described what happened after births at home:

> The mother was an active participant rather than being passively processed.
> She picked up her baby immediately after birth rather than having it handed to
> her. She stroked the baby's face with her fingertips and then started to move her
> whole palm over the baby's body and head in just a few minutes, whereas
> mothers in hospital usually take much longer to move from the first tentative
> finger-tip touching as if stroking a very fragile object to the whole-palm contact
> typical of home deliveries.[2]

Everyone present became excited and the mother often almost
ectastic. Macfarlane's videotapes of labour in hospital[3] show that the
setting of the birth and the people assisting affect this mood considerably.
Though some midwives and doctors share in creating the same elevated
mood, others seem to dampen enthusiasm and loving interaction. The
presence of the husband or other partner may also be significant in the
expression of spontaneous emotions.

At home everybody in the room looks at the newborn baby for
prolonged periods. In hospital, on the contrary, the baby is often put in a
crib and is only intermittently looked at while the team gets on with the
third stage of labour and the suturing. At home the mother is groomed,
in the sense that those present brush her hair, wash her face, change her
clothes, help her put a flower in her nightdress or a ribbon in her hair,
while at the same time offering evidence of joy and affection by cuddling,
kissing, or stroking the new mother, patting her on the head or holding
her hand, depending on the relationship with her. Behaviour tends to be
much more muted after many hospital deliveries and in some all
behaviour of this kind is noticeably lacking.

At home the baby is put to the breast within 6 minutes or so, and
precedes suckling by licking the nipple for a long time. In hospital the
baby may not be put to the breast for several hours or more, and then it is
often supposed to 'get on with it and no nonsense', the midwife or nurse

---

[1] J. H. Kennell, M. A. Tause, and M. H. Klaus: Evidence for a sensitive period in
the human mother. *Parent – infant interaction*. CIBA Foundation Symposium 33
(1975).
[2] Quoted in Rubin Chec: Maternal touch. *Child and Family* 4, (1965).
[3] Aidan Macfarlane: *The psychology of childbirth*. Fontana, London (1977).

The baby born at home

standing over the mother and if she thinks necessary holding the baby's head against the breast.[1]

Finally at home both parents tend to talk to the baby in high-pitched voices, spontaneously choosing a level which is the easiest for the newborn baby to hear,[2] whereas in hospital as we have seen, no one may be talking to the baby at all.

In a retrospective study of 266 deliveries by Donald Garrow and Diana Smith,[3] of which 26 were at home, 31 per cent of the mothers delivered in hospital did not hold their babies for several hours or even days after birth whereas all but one of the mothers delivered at home held their babies within the first hour.

In the United States Marshall Klaus revealed that in 1400 premature nurseries in 1970 only 34 per cent let mothers handle their babies.[4]

Changes have now been made in many hospitals and there is a new awareness in special-care baby-units of the importance of mothers being able to see, touch, hold when possible, and help care for their babies. But in many hospitals, both in the nursery and on the wards, the environment provided interferes with the development of a personal relationship between mother and newborn, tends to distort the mother's interpretation of her baby's needs, and often saps her confidence.[5] This can have far-reaching consequences. Research with mothers who have been battering their babies shows that a much larger proportion of these mothers have been separated from these particular babies following delivery as compared with other children they did not harm.[6]

Mothers themselves know that it is often extraordinarily difficult to relate to a baby who is in special care or who is separated from the mother in the first days after birth. I have had many letters from and talked with a large number of women who have suffered from being emotionally 'frozen' towards a particular child who was taken away from them following delivery. They are anxious about this, resentful of the child, and guilty because of their own hostile feelings.

But a woman can be separated from her baby even if it is by her bed if

[1] Sheila Kitzinger: *The experience of breastfeeding,* op. cit.
[2] C. and S. J. Hutt: Auditory discrimination at birth in *Early human development* (ed. S. J. and C. Hutt), Oxford University Press (1973).
[3] The modern practice of separating a new-born baby from its mother, *Proceedings of the Royal Society of Medicine* **69**, 22 – 5 (1976).
[4] J. H. Kennell *et al., Parent – infant interaction,* op. cit.
[5] Sheila Kitzinger: *The good birth guide.* op. cit.
[6] M. A. Lynch: Ill health and child abuse, *Lancet* **ii**, 317 (1975).

such strong drugs for pain relief have been used in labour that not only the mother is drowsy and not interested in her baby, but the baby is unresponsive too. It is very difficult to work up any lasting interest in a baby who rarely opens its eyes, who is floppy, and who does not suck well. Chemical separation can interfere with mother – baby interaction as completely as physical separation.[1,2] Pethidine can affect the baby for more than a month[3] and reduce interaction between mother and baby for a year or longer.[4] It is often claimed that epidurals do not affect the baby at all. *All* anaesthesia enters the mother's and hence the baby's blood stream. Regional anaesthesia tends to produce babies who at 3 days old are irritable with decreased muscle tone. This may not matter much in terms of the baby's health, but it must affect the relationship between mother and baby.[5]

Donald Garrow and Diana Smith, writing from the point of view of paediatrics, say:

We believe that the best place for a normal woman to be delivered is in her own home. . . . Birth at home is an exciting family affair, whereas in hospital (although it may be exciting and happy) labour is too often reduced to a series of technical procedures. Exciting events make a deep impression and aid the attachment process.

At home the relationship between mother and baby has the best chance of starting off from the first moments of life as a going concern.

[1] D. M. Smith and D. H. Garrow: *The place of birth,* op. cit.
[2] T. B. Brazelton: Effect of pre-natal drugs on the behavior of the neonate, *American Journal of Psychiatry* **126**, 1261 – 6 (1970).
[3] E. Conway and Y. Brackbill: Delivery, medication and infant outcome, *Monograph of Society for Research on Child Development,* **35**, 24 – 34 (1970).
[4] Martin Richards: The one-day-old deprived child, *New Scientist,* March 1974.
[5] D. H. Garrow and D. M. Smith, *The place of birth,* op. cit.

5

Arranging a home birth

WOMEN who hope to deliver at home have to be very certain that this is what they want and to start arrangements for it early in pregnancy. Of 65 women who had home births whose experiences I studied[1] all but a few had encountered difficulty in obtaining a home birth and many obstacles had been put in their way to try to prevent them. 'I was appalled to find that there were absolutely no facilities for home delivery in our area', one woman wrote. 'A fruitless search for a friendly doctor or midwife drew a complete blank.' This couple went on and delivered the baby themselves. Another couple kept a diary describing their experiences of trying to get a home birth; in the end they were successful, but it took them 4 months before arrangements could be made and the uncertainty of where the birth was to take place made the mother anxious during much of her pregnancy.

One mother who wrote that she felt she had to 'fight' for a home birth until 2 weeks before she had the baby said that her doctor refused to do a home delivery because he told her that 'my place on the .... Committee would be in jeopardy' and 'If you have a home delivery, everyone'll want one'. Yet another mother wrote:

Home deliveries are virtually 'verboten' here. Nonetheless my husband and I felt absolutely unequivocally that the most suitable place for our baby to be introduced to this planet was in our own home, unless, of course, there was a very good reason to have hospital care. None of the local GPs was prepared to take me on, and we were eventually summoned to see the chief obstetrician of the area, who underlined that a home delivery was out of the question. Not surprised at this, we politely said that we should have been very grateful for expert assistance at the delivery, but, since this was not to be forthcoming, we preferred to take our chances on our own at home. Several weeks later, quite out of the blue, a letter arrived, informing us that three midwives had been assigned to me, and thereafter they took

[1] Sheila Kitzinger and John Davis (Eds.): *The place of birth*. Oxford University Press (1978),

care of me at home. ... The midwives were super ladies, not least because
they accepted our right to have a say in the matter.

A spokesman for the Royal College of Midwives states that: 'The
difficulty is not a shortage of midwives as much as a shortage of
GPs willing to be on call during a home birth. Some midwives are
already handling home deliveries without backing from a GP,
relying on a flying squad from a hospital if anything goes wrong.'[1]

Britain has a rate of almost 100 per cent hospital deliveries today.
In 1965 40 per cent of births took place at home or in small
maternity homes outside the National Health Service. By 1974 that
figure was down to 6 per cent[2] and by 1976 there was a further
decline to less than 3 per cent. Some areas have no facilities at all
for home births and anyone wanting one in those parts of the
country has to be prepared to go outside the system. Other areas,
like Oxford and East Anglia, have maintained the option of home
birth and have a very low perinatal mortality rate. (Oxford and
East Anglia are two of the safest places in the country to have a
baby whether it is born in hospital or at home.)

The run-down of the domiciliary services is largely the result of
the Cranbrook Committee's report in 1959. The Committee studied
the organizational changes which they considered necessary in the
maternity services and recommended that home births should be
reduced to 30 per cent of all deliveries. But once the hospital beds
were created (and they were increased annually between 1967 and
1971) home births dropped to well below this figure, partly because
new maternity units had been built and old ones enlarged to cope
with what was in 1958 a rapidly expanding birth rate, and when the
birth rate declined from the mid-1960s until 1977 the hospital beds
were still there. In 1978 there was evidence of an increase of 7000
births. The girls born in the early 1960s had reached childbearing
age. This halt in the steady decline of the previous 13 years may
mean that more options about the place of birth are available to
women.

In spite of the steady phasing out of home births the Department
of Health and Social Security states that 'it has never been our
intention that health authorities should refuse a home confinement

[1] Moira Brown, quoted in *General Practitioner* 3 March 1978.
[2] Eva Alberman in *Benefits and hazards of the new obstetrics* (ed. Tim Chard and
Martin Richards). Heinemann, London (1977).

to a woman who wishes to have one'[1], that it 'does not expect
pressure to be placed upon the woman to accept hospital
confinement against her express wishes'[2] and that it is willing to
look into complaints from those who are having difficulties in
getting a doctor or midwife to attend a home birth. David Ennals,
Minister of Health, answering a question in parliament.[3], said that
if a woman chose home delivery 'health authorities should ensure
that the services necessary to make home delivery as safe as possible
are provided'. Going into hospital to have a baby, although it may
be advised, is not compulsory for anyone.

If you think you would like to have your baby at home the first
person to talk to is your doctor, whom you may find understanding
and helpful. Many doctors believe, however, that *all* babies should
be born in hospital. It is reasonable to expect, therefore, that they
will try to dissuade you from having a home birth, and some may
tell you that you are risking your baby's life. (Birth can never be
100 per cent safe, and of course some babies die wherever they are
born, usually because they are of very low birth weight.)

Since you may feel especially vulnerable and emotional when
discussing this subject with the doctor it is a good idea to have your
husband present and to write down the advice you are given so that
you can think about it cooly afterwards. You do not have to come
to snap decisions, but can say, 'We'd like time to think this over
and talk about it together'.

The doctor's professional responsibility means that he or she
cannot make firm promises about home birth in early pregnancy
when it cannot yet be known if all will be well in five or six months'
time. Most GPs who agree to one will only do so provided the
pregnancy is straightforward.

The *general practitioner obstetrician* to whom you go for
maternity care need not be your usual GP, and you can ask to have
maternity care from another GP. There is often only one partner in
a practice who does maternity work anyway, so you may *have* to go
to another doctor during pregnancy. This will normally be
arranged by your present GP. But if you are thinking of a home
birth, it is worth asking the GP *as soon as pregnancy is diagnosed*
(because you then have time in which to explore all the alternatives)

---

[1] Letter to Society to Support Home Confinements (12 July 1976).
[2] Letter to Society to Support Home Confinements (17 September 1976).
[3] Reported in *General Practitioner,* 3 March 1978.

if his or her partner is prepared to do home deliveries provided everything is likely to be straightforward, and if not whether you can have the name of a GP obstetrician who is. Remember that many young doctors have never seen a home confinement and so may not have the confidence to do one, and that many older ones have had little practice over the last few years.

Should your own doctor not know of a GP who does home confinements, you may wish to ring up or write to the *Area Nursing Officer* (look in the phone book for your city or county health Department) and ask for the names of GPs on the Obstetric List who sometimes do home confinements. You will probably be put in touch with the Community Nursing Officer who supervises the community midwives (those who do deliveries in the GP unit and also occasionally at home). If you have already decided that you want to have your baby at home, let her know that you feel strongly about it, and ask how midwifery cover can be arranged. She is likely to understand how you feel and may herself enjoy home deliveries.

If you find that you meet a dead end, write explaining what has happened to your *Community Health Council*; say that you still feel strongly that you want to have a home birth, and ask them if they can help. You may like to send copies of your letter to the Area Nursing Officer and to the Family Practitioner Committee, the address of which you can get from the Health Department. *According to her conditions of service, established by the Central Midwives Board, a midwife called when you are in labour at home must attend.*

If you already have a GP obstetrician who is opposed to home birth or if you are attending a Consultant Unit but want to have a home birth instead, it is probably best to put your reasons for wanting one in writing to the doctor concerned and the Area Nursing Officer. Try to be very clear and unemotional about it. It is important that your husband agrees with you and a good idea to sign the letter jointly. As with all correspondence about the place of birth, keep a copy of your letter, and the reply. If your reason for wanting a home birth is because you want to avoid going into a particular hospital, explain in detail why it is that you do not want to go into hospital.

If you have decided on a home birth, the midwife attached to the practice will come and look at your home to see whether it is suitable and easy for her to get to, and to advise you what to do to

66

make everything ready. It is expected that there should be running water and that the place is clean and convenient, but there is no need to try to reproduce hospital conditions in the home.

As the estimated date approaches, she will leave a sterile maternity pack in your home. All that you will need to provide is a bucket and a few bowls and things which most households have already. There is usually no need to re-arrange the bedroom, though it is easier if the bed is at right angles to the wall.

The midwife will ask you who is going to housekeep and look after you in the week after the birth, as you should have ample opportunity to rest.

Social services departments have a statutory duty to provide home helps after home confinements for a period of 14 days. If the GP considers that help is necessary for a longer period and informs the department, the home help can continue for longer.

Useful addreses for further information about home birth in Britain are:

The National Childbirth Trust, 9 Queensborough Terrace, Bayswater, London, W2;

The Birth Centre, 188 Old Street, London, EC1 (telephone 01-251 0768, 2 – 4 p.m.);

The Association for the Improvement of the Maternity Services, West Hill Cottage, Exmouth Place, Hastings, Sussex TN34 3JA (Secretary: Anne Taylor);

The Society to Support Home Confinements, Margaret Whyte, 17 Laburnum Avenue, Durham City.

In the United States and Canada the situation is radically different in different states. There is a severe shortage of trained nurse midwives able to take responsibility for home births and licensed to attend them and, unfortunately, no obstetric flying squad service. In some states although midwives are available they are not allowed to do deliveries or to be present at a birth, except in emergencies, without the attendance of an obstetrician or they lose their licences. Further information about the state of affairs in various states and cities can be obtained from:

The National Association of Parents and Professionals for Safe Alternatives in Childbirth (NAPSAC), PO Box 267, Marble Hill, Missouri 63764;

Birth at home

from the local chapter of the International Childbirth Education Association, PO Box 20852, Milwaukee, Wisconsin 53220;

or from the American Society for Psychoprophylaxis in Obstetrics, 1411 K Street, N.W., Washington DC 20005.

The Practising Midwife (this is a midwifery journal), 156 Drakes Lane, Summertown, Tennessee 38483
may be able to tell you of an empirical midwife in your area. It is, however, very important to find one who is highly experienced and responsible and works closely with an obstetrician should a doctor's help or hospital admission be needed.

The Association for Childbirth at Home International, Box 1219, Cerritos, California 90701
have their own certified childbirth educators and a training course for those planning home birth.

Other addresses with people who may be able to help are:

Alternative Birth Center, 5 Warren Square, Jamaica Plain, Massachusetts 02130;

American College of Home Obstetrics, Suite 600, 664 North Michigan Avenue, Chicago, Illinois 60611 (information about doctors doing home deliveries);

Association for Childbirth Alternatives, San Luis Obispo, California;

Better Alternatives Birth Information, Education and Services, 1941 Strand, Missoula, Montana 59801;

Birth Alternatives, 43 Clover Lane, Princeton, New Jersey 08540;

Cooperative Childbirth Network, 14 Truesdale Drive, Croton-on-Hudson, NY 10520;

Family Health Center, 2522 Dana Street, Suite 201, Berkeley, California 94704;

Home Oriented Maternity Experience, 511 New York Avenue, Takoma Park, Washington DC 20012;

Informed Homebirth, P.O. Box 788, Boulder, Colorado 80306;

Maternity Center Association, Bethesda, Maryland 20014;

The Midwife and the Doctor, Homecover, RFD3, Putney, Vermont 05436;

Midwife to Midwife, RD2, Box 140, Bristol, Vermont 05443 (an organisation for midwives);

Mountain People's Clinic, Hayesville, North Carolina;

National Midwives Association, Maternity Center, 1119 East San Antonio Avenue, El Paso, Texas 79901;

New York Home Coming Clinic, 4521 20th Street, New York;

University of Missouri Women's Center;

Arranging a home birth

Womancare, Women's Health Center, San Diego, California;
The Women's Alternative Health Clinic, 70 Central Avenue, Wailuku, Hawaii 96793.

Women's Health Groups and Alternative Birth Centers are increasing at such a rate that by the time this is printed there will be many more. These are simply those of which I know. This is by no means an exhaustive list, but one or other of these organizations will be able to put an enquirer in touch with one near her own home. Find out exactly what they offer, the training and experience birth assistants have, and talk with couples who have had babies with them and where possible compare options, before you make up your mind.

Education for birth

Anyone planning a home birth would do well to attend childbirth education classes, and try to find those which are for couples, not only for expectant mothers. In Britain these can be discovered through the National Childbirth Trust, 9 Queensborough Terrace, Bayswater, London, W2.

In the United States ASPO and ICEA and the Association for Home Oriented Birth Experience and Husband-Coached Childbirth all run classes. The addresses of the first three are on p. 68 and the address of the latter, which teaches the Bradley method, is P.O. Box 5224, Sherman Oaks, California 01413.

In Canada the Canadian Childbirth Education Association will be able to let you know of classes near you. Write to CEA of Toronto, 33 Price Street, Toronto, Ontario M4W 1Z2.

In Australia write to The Childbirth Education Association of Australia, Box N206, Grosvenor Street P.O., Sydney, New South Wales 2000; The Australian Birth Foundation, 116 Glenferrie Road, (P.O. Box 133), Malvern, Victoria 3144; or Parents Centres Australia, 148 Hereford Street, Forest Lodge, NSW 2037. The Australian Birth Foundation, 116 Glenferrie Road, Malvern, Victoria 3144 and the Childbirth and Parenthood Association of Western Australia, 19 Croydon Street, Nedlands, Western Australia 6009 may also be able to help.

In New Zealand contact Parents Centre Federation, P.O. Box 29 094, Fendalton, Christchurch.

Birth at home

In South Africa ask the Paramedical Association for Childbirth Education, 6 Scott Street, Waverley, 2001 Johannesburg.

My book on preparation for birth, *The experience of childbirth,* will I hope also be of help to you. There are also cassette tapes, *Journey through birth,* in which I talk directly to the couple practising for birth and teach breathing and relaxation. These are obtainable in Britain from the NCT and in the USA from The ICEA Bookstore, P.O. Box 70258, Seattle, Washington 98107.

Couples having a baby at home need classes which are highly informative and which offer a depth of understanding which the woman who is relying on others to get her baby born for her may not require. Classes should last two hours or so and the course should consist of at least six sessions, with plenty of opportunity for questions and free discussion. There should be specific instruction for birth partners and their role during the labour, both about what is happening physiologically, how it may feel to the woman in labour at different phases, and how a partner can help. There should be detailed teaching about variations in kinds of labour, how to cope with back-ache labour, for instance, and about the things that most usually make labour difficult and how the woman can be helped to handle pain and discomfort. Health, sensible living and relaxation in pregnancy and emotional aspects of preparation for birth, the experience of labour, and the postpartum days, should all be fully discussed. Classes geared exclusively to hospital delivery are not suitable for those having their babies at home, and it is important that a teacher be found who has knowledge of what is entailed in home birth and who is psychologically supportive.

Anyone attending the birth should understand what the woman has learned and have basic knowledge about the different kinds of breathing, techniques of relaxation, positions the woman may like to get into, massage that may help, other comfort techniques which her partner may use and, most important, the words and phrases which are most meaningful for her in stimulating her to respond appropriately to contractions and to different stressful physical sensations such as pressure of the foetal head against the rectum and anus.

Equipment useful for a home birth

There should be a car available (with plenty of petrol) to take the mother to hospital if necessary. In Britain the midwife will either take the mother in her own car or call the ambulance if she needs to be moved.

There should be a phone, either in the home or by arrangement available at a neighbour's house. A list of important phone numbers (the midwife, the doctor, hospital, etc.) should be stuck or pinned near it.

Running water, preferably on the same floor as the birth room, is necessary and a lavatory as near the birth room as possible. The birth room does not have to be the bedroom. An electric kettle, so that water can be boiled in the birth room, is useful, even if it is only used for filling a hot-water bottle and making tea.

Although some women like to labour on a mattress on the floor, this can be hard on a midwife's back if she is not accustomed to sitting on the floor. Probably most women deliver in bed, but the mattress should be firm. A rubber sheet should be put on the bed a couple of weeks before the birth is due in case the waters break at night. A *chaise longue* (a settee the end of which is open at both sides) is sometimes convenient as it allows the mother to sit up well supported and there is space at the bottom for the birth attendant to sit at the time of delivery. Two bean bags, covered in material which can be wiped or washed, can be excellent. The mother can sit on one and have the other behind her for back support. They provide a firm base and a flat, hard surface. They can be used on the floor or if it is more comfortable for the midwife they can be put on the bed. Other kinds of cushioned support for the labouring woman can be provided by foam wedges like those often used in childbirth education classes. A special back support consisting of two kinds of foam moulded to the curve of a pregnant women's back at term (Fig. 2) and covered in towelling is also available (Fig. 3) and although it would be expensive for one family to use, could be hired out by a Birth Centre or other organization. It is called the Kitzinger Cushion, is available from Sylvester Furniture, Little Clarendon Street, Oxford, and costs £35 plus VAT and postage.

Extra pillows are always useful.

One great advantage of a home birth is that you do not have to go to bed until you feel like it and provided that you have a convenient alternative place in which to deliver, you need not go to bed at all.

As we saw in Chapter 2, lying flat on a bed is now thought to be a

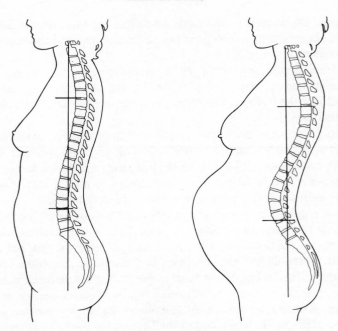

FIG. 2. The change in the curve of the lower spine in late pregnancy

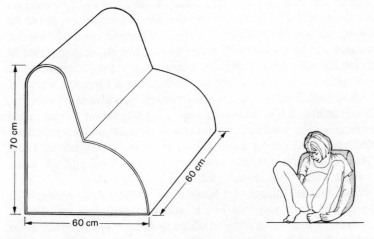

FIG. 3. The Kitzinger cushion

One comfortable position for bearing down

72

major cause of reduced trans-placental blood flow to the baby. It can also result in drastically lowered blood-pressure in the mother which makes her feel sick, giddy, and faint. This is because in late pregnancy when a woman lies on her back her heavy, enlarged uterus presses against both the inferior vena cava and the lower aorta (see p. 19).

When planning for a home birth think about all the comfortable seating, forms of back support, and activities which you may enjoy which will both allow blood to flow readily across the placenta and also help the descent of the baby's head by letting gravity work.

A woman who has a backache labour, which often occurs when the baby is posterior (facing towards her front rather than towards her back) will not be comfortable sitting up or in any position in which she puts weight on her spine. She will also appreciate her back being rubbed or having firm pressure applied to it from the heel of the palm or the knuckles of an assistant. So she may be most comfortable on all fours or kneeling well forward, supported by a bean bag underneath her. Alternatively large floor cushions can be heaped to make a suitable base and covered with a clean sheet, but they are more difficult to mould into shapes which are retained.

Extra heating should be available in a form which allows the temperature of the birth room to be increased speedily just before delivery if it is a cold day, so that the baby is delivered into a warm atmosphere. If it is very hot weather, an electric fan is useful.

There should be efficient lighting, but not lighting which shines in the labouring woman's eyes. A flexible stemmed lamp is necessary so that very good light can be directed onto the perineum in the second stage of labour. All lights can usually be dimmed once the baby is born and beathing well.

It is easiest to have all small equipment which might be needed for the birth on a small table or trolley beside the mother. Rest everything on a clean, ironed cloth and cover it with another. Some things can be kept covered in plastic bags until they are needed.

In Britain the midwife will provide all the sterile equipment necessary and leaves a pack at the home some time before the baby is due. When this is not done, however, these things have to be provided. They include a thick paper pad to cover and protect the mattress. Thick pads made out of newspapers, with an old cotton sheet put over that work well. The kind of large soft paper pads lined with plastic which are used by people who are incontinent, or disposable nappies, are useful for sitting on and may be enough.

If the midwife is not providing a sterile pack and other equipment you may also need:

Shoe laces or narrow tape for tying the cord, should be boiled before use. The cord is tied or clamped in two places and a cut made between them.

A thermometer. The mother's temperature should be taken a few hours after the birth and again twice a day for the first 3 days, and thereafter once a day. A rise in temperature is likely to occur if she gets engorged as the milk comes in on the third or fourth day, but it might also mean that there is some infection. If it does not go down as soon as the engorgement is dealt with by expression of milk, feeding the baby and cold compresses on the breasts,it should be reported to the doctor.

Some cotton swabs, which can be baked ready in a clean biscuit tin in an oven at 250°F for 1 hour. These are useful for wiping the baby's face after delivery if it needs washing, and for gently cleaning the cord stump when necessary.

The cardboard cylinder from a lavatory paper roll lets the father hear the foetal heart. Tonya Brooks and Linda Bennett of the Association for Childbirth at Home International, recommend a 'metal double-shot jigger with hole punched through center'[1] (a jigger is used for measuring out spirits) but the midwife should bring a stethoscope with her.

Antiseptic solution, preferably of a kind that does not sting sore perineal tissues. Washing the perineum is best done by using boiled, cooled water in a jug to which a little antiseptic has been added and then pouring it over the perineum. Do not use swabs or a facecloth. A bidet is even better.

A large Pyrex or other easily cleaned bowl to receive the placenta. Another smaller bowl or jam jar to hold antiseptic solution with thermometer and scissors for cutting the cord.

A graded jug for measuring blood loss following delivery.

Pedal-bin plastic liners or other disposable waste bags are useful for soiled pads.

[1] *Giving birth at home,* the parent information booklet of ACH (1976).

Arranging a home birth

The largest size sanitary pads are the best for the first few days after delivery, and since they should be changed frequently 4 packets may be required. A belt to keep pads in position.

Suppositories or disposable enema, to be used only if necessary.

Clock or watch with second hand with which to time contractions and work out the rate of the foetal heart. It should be between 120 and 160 beats per minute. Time for 15 seconds and multiply by 4.

Ice cube chips for the mother to suck during labour.

Two small, real sponges, obtainable from artists' shops, which can be dipped in iced water and used to refresh the mother.

Bucket over which the mother can squat to pass urine during labour. She should empty her bladder every hour to hour and a half.

A facecloth.

Hairbrush, ribbons, or something suitable for keeping her hair out of the way if she has long hair and gets hot.

A small gardening spray such as is used for window boxes or green plants which is filled with ice-cold water and used to refresh the mother's face. Alternatively Evian water is sold in aerosol form and in France orange flower water in an aerosol container is very refreshing, or get orange flower water from the chemist's and put it in a garden spray.

A camera if you want to take photographs.

Tape recorder or record player if you may like music during labour.

Flowers, a painting, or anything beautiful the mother may like to focus on during difficult contractions.

A hot-water bottle, or plastic-covered heating pad (it may get damp) in case the mother gets cold. Useful for her feet or against her back.

Two or three picnic ice-packs, one semi-frozen in case a cold stimulus feels right (e.g. to relieve backache) and a hot one, warmed in a pan of hot water, to take the place of a hot water bottle in the small of the back, over the lower uterus, or between the top of the legs.

Birth at home

Honey for early labour if things start slowly. A laid tray and raspberry-leaf tea (this can be bought at Health Food Stores) or other tea for sipping. A few lemons and a squeezer for making a lemon and water iced drink. Sustaining food for any labour assistants. Celebratory food and drink for after the birth.

Talcum powder to sprinkle lightly on skin which is being massaged.

A soft towel or small flanelette sheet in which to wrap the baby.

Something warm and light to throw over mother and baby after delivery. A continental quilt is ideal. The area of greatest heat loss is the baby's head; a quilt can be tucked round the head so that the baby stays snug.

Clean sheets for making up the bed afresh.

Towels, soap.

Something in which to weigh the baby.

But more important than any of these things is a *peaceful, calm, unhurried atmosphere.*

It is useful to have an exercise book in which to keep a log of labour. Divide it into columns, with one for the time, one for description of what has happened physiologically, i.e. the duration of contractions and interval between them, dilatation of the cervix, the foetal heart rate, when the mother has emptied her bladder, her pulse and blood pressure, a note of when the membranes rupture, when the second stage starts and so on.

In one column note what the mother is doing to handle this phase of her labour and how she feels. Indicate her subjective experience of contractions, sensations of pressure and fullness, pain, stretching, sleepiness, energy, etc. The mother herself may like to keep this log in the earlier part of the first stage, the father then taking over. They will both be so busy during the second stage that this will probably have to be written up immediately after the birth. But the log will mean that there is a complete record of the birth. If labour starts slowly it is easy to forget what happened and when in describing to midwife or doctor what occurred several hours before, and the log book also means that the parents can provide accurate information about the progress in the first part of the first stage whether or not a baby is born at home.

Arranging a home birth

After the birth eau-de-cologne, deodorants, clean nightdresses help the mother to feel fresh. She may feel ravenously hungry and thirsty, so plenty of fluids and nourishing food should be quickly available.

Your parents

Unless the relations with parents are very easy and you feel the same way about baby care and feeding it is probably best not to accept an offer from a prospective grandmother to stay around the time of the birth or afterwards. New parents are in a stressed state, even though excited and happy, and it is not the best time to face the challenge of difficult relationships. One is also less likely to be considerate and thoughtful about other people's needs when caught up in the tide of strong emotions. A couple need time alone together with their baby to get to know each other and especially after the first birth to feel their way into the role of parents and the changed relationship between them. Because even if you hope that nothing will change and that you can go on as before, in fact your whole life-style is bound to be affected, and you will find that your interests tend to become baby-centred at least for a time and that you have a new sense of the other partner as a father or mother rather than only a husband or wife. Many of the things to be discovered about each other and yourself then are positive and enriching; others may be disturbing at first and require some emotional adjustment.

Each new mother also has to find her own way with her baby in an intimate personal relationship and other people's advice is usually not helpful. Even *feeling* that your mother disapproves at the number of times you are feeding or the way you handle the baby can introduce tension into the interaction with her. And the grandmother who is determined not to interfere but wants to help may go to bed at night and in spite of her own good intentions lie awake worrying about what her daughter is doing to the baby, or about your marriage or mental stability. So it is probably wiser to have parents to stay when you are over the first period of adaptation to the baby and have settled into parenthood with some confidence.

This is why the best solution to having enough help is for the husband to take a week or two off work and arrange for occasional

TABLE 6

Birth at home

January / *October* → *November*
1 2 3 4 5 6 7 8 9 10 11 12 13 14 15 16 17 18 19 20 21 22 23 24 25 26 27 28 29 30 31
8 9 10 11 12 13 14 15 16 17 18 19 20 21 22 23 24 25 26 27 28 29 30 31 1 2 3 4 5 6 7

February / *November* → *December*
1 2 3 4 5 6 7 8 9 10 11 12 13 14 15 16 17 18 19 20 21 22 23 24 25 26 27 28
8 9 10 11 12 13 14 15 16 17 18 19 20 21 22 23 24 25 26 27 28 29 30 1 2 3 4 5

March / *December* → *January*
1 2 3 4 5 6 7 8 9 10 11 12 13 14 15 16 17 18 19 20 21 22 23 24 25 26 27 28 29 30 31
6 7 8 9 10 11 12 13 14 15 16 17 18 19 20 21 22 23 24 25 26 27 28 29 30 31 1 2 3 4 5

April / *January* → *February*
1 2 3 4 5 6 7 8 9 10 11 12 13 14 15 16 17 18 19 20 21 22 23 24 25 26 27 28 29 30
6 7 8 9 10 11 12 13 14 15 16 17 18 19 20 21 22 23 24 25 26 27 28 29 30 31 1 2 3 4

May / *February* → *March*
1 2 3 4 5 6 7 8 9 10 11 12 13 14 15 16 17 18 19 20 21 22 23 24 25 26 27 28 29 30 31
5 6 7 8 9 10 11 12 13 14 15 16 17 18 19 20 21 22 23 24 25 26 27 28 1 2 3 4 5 6 7

June / *March* → *April*
1 2 3 4 5 6 7 8 9 10 11 12 13 14 15 16 17 18 19 20 21 22 23 24 25 26 27 28 29 30
8 9 10 11 12 13 14 15 16 17 18 19 20 21 22 23 24 25 26 27 28 29 30 31 1 2 3 4 5 6

July / *April* → *May*
1 2 3 4 5 6 7 8 9 10 11 12 13 14 15 16 17 18 19 20 21 22 23 24 25 26 27 28 29 30 31
7 8 9 10 11 12 13 14 15 16 17 18 19 20 21 22 23 24 25 26 27 28 29 30 1 2 3 4 5 6 7

August / *May* → *June*
1 2 3 4 5 6 7 8 9 10 11 12 13 14 15 16 17 18 19 20 21 22 23 24 25 26 27 28 29 30 31
8 9 10 11 12 13 14 15 16 17 18 19 20 21 22 23 24 25 26 27 28 29 30 31 1 2 3 4 5 6 7

September / *June* → *July*
1 2 3 4 5 6 7 8 9 10 11 12 13 14 15 16 17 18 19 20 21 22 23 24 25 26 27 28 29 30
8 9 10 11 12 13 14 15 16 17 18 19 20 21 22 23 24 25 26 27 28 29 30 1 2 3 4 5 6 7

October / *July* → *August*
1 2 3 4 5 6 7 8 9 10 11 12 13 14 15 16 17 18 19 20 21 22 23 24 25 26 27 28 29 30 31
8 9 10 11 12 13 14 15 16 17 18 19 20 21 22 23 24 25 26 27 28 29 30 31 1 2 3 4 5 6 7

November / *August* → *September*
1 2 3 4 5 6 7 8 9 10 11 12 13 14 15 16 17 18 19 20 21 22 23 24 25 26 27 28 29 30
8 9 10 11 12 13 14 15 16 17 18 19 20 21 22 23 24 25 26 27 28 29 30 31 1 2 3 4 5 6

December / *September* → *October*
1 2 3 4 5 6 7 8 9 10 11 12 13 14 15 16 17 18 19 20 21 22 23 24 25 26 27 28 29 30 31
7 8 9 10 11 12 13 14 15 16 17 18 19 20 21 22 23 24 25 26 27 28 29 30 1 2 3 4 5 6 7

78

absences after that time if at all possible.

I believe that we should create a new institution, the *babymoon,* equivalent to a honeymoon, for both parents to start the relationship with their new baby.[1]

Working out when the baby is due

In the upper horizontal row of numbers in Table 6, find the first day of your last period; the number beneath, set in italics, will show the end of 280 days or ten months of 28 days each. This gives you the estimated date of delivery (EDD).

---

[1] For discussion of the emotional work to be done, see Sheila Kitzinger: *The experience of breastfeeding, Penguin, Harmondsworth (1979).*

6

Drugs and diet
in pregnancy

THOSE who see childbirth primarily as a medical event put major emphasis on obstetric intervention at the time of labour. Those who see it as a significant psychological and social experience and a process in which the woman accepts responsibility for her own body put emphasis on the prevention of disease and malfunction through healthy living and the maintenance of the optimal conditions for mother and baby throughout pregnancy. The woman and her unborn child are in a partnership for nine months. Regular antenatal visits, though very important, cannot ensure that the environment in which the foetus is growing is not adversely affected by pollutants. Toxic substances from the environment in which the mother lives, the food she eats, the air she breathes, the drugs she takes, and the anxiety and fear she may experience may all affect that partnership in some way.

The woman who wants to retain her autonomy over the processes of childbearing should look at her environment and at the way in which she lives, even before conception, to see how she can create the conditions which give her and her baby the best possible basis for birth at home. She has the right to have her baby at home if she wishes. She also has the responsibility during pregnancy to provide her baby with the best chance to start life whole and healthy, and a responsibility to herself, too, to care for her body and to begin motherhood full of vitality. Nobody can do this for her.

The following section is, I realize, not a comforting one. Read it in broad daylight, and at the *beginning,* not the end of pregnancy.

Drugs in pregnancy

No pregnant woman should smoke. Smoking is dangerous not only for the mother's health, but for the baby. When a pregnant woman smokes she forces toxic substances into the foetal blood stream, and the spontaneous respiratory movements with which the baby rehearses the actions which after birth will become breathing are interrupted. In effect, the baby coughs and splutters. The foetal heart rate also speeds up and the baby often starts to move about. It is interesting that this effect on the heart rate often occurs even before the mother lights up, in response to anticipation of the event.[1]

British statistics indicate that smoking after the fourth month of pregnancy reduces the newborn baby's birth weight by on average 6 ozs (170 g). This does not mean that every woman who smokes gives birth to an underweight baby. I have known heavy smokers announce triumphantly that their babies were 7½ lbs (3.4 kg) as if they had proved a point against the statisticians. But it does mean that women who smoke tend to push their babies into the low birth-weight and hence high-risk category. But it is not just a question of the baby being small. Smoking increases the risk of the baby being still-born or dying shortly after birth by about a quarter. The National Child Development Study followed 1500 children from birth till they were eleven. Those born to mothers who smoked 10 or more cigarettes a day during pregnancy were on average 3 – 5 months behind in reading, mathematics, and general abilities compared with the children of non-smoking mothers.

Women intending to have a home birth should not smoke and if they have smoked in early pregnancy should give it up if possible by the fourth month, when the effect on the baby is likely to be minimal.

There are women who just have to smoke if they are not to become so tense that life becomes intolerable. Anxiety about smoking can actually increase their desire to smoke. If a pregnant woman has got into this state it is probably best to ration herself to a few pleasurable cigarettes a day and allow herself to really enjoy them. But she would be wise to consider a hospital rather than a home delivery.

When a woman intends to give up smoking it is only fair for her partner and anyone else in the immediate family with whom she is in regular contact to give it up at the same time.

[1] M. Ottariano *et al.*: On the effects of smoke on foetal health, paper given at 5th International Congress of Psychosomatic Obstetrics and Gynaecology, Rome (1977).

Drugs and diet in pregnancy

Cannabis has not been adequately researched because mothers who smoke it during pregnancy are unlikely to admit they do lest legal action is taken. It is widely used, however, and in some American communes is thought to help relaxation and peace of mind during pregnancy. I have had mothers attending childbirth education classes who have smoked it during labour. If a mother feels she has to smoke something cannabis may be safer than ordinary tobacco. But since we know so little about its effects on the baby it cannot be recommended.

Recently it has been suggested that both tea and coffee may be harmful. Here again, evidence is slight, and what there is suggests that a woman would have to drink between 10 and 20 cups a day to risk damaging a baby, consuming a total of 30 – 60 mg/kg of body weight of caffeine.[1] In fact no caffeine-related teratogenic effects have been reported in human beings, though they do occur in mice.

Alcohol, however, is potentially toxic to the foetus. We do not yet know if there is a safe level of alcohol consumption during pregnancy. Many women come to dislike alcohol in early pregnancy and spontaneously avoid it. They often tolerate it better and enjoy an occasional drink in the middle and third trimesters and there is no evidence that their babies come to any harm from moderate drinking of this kind. (I spent a marvellous few days wine-tasting in the Moselle a week before our first child was born.) However, it is now known that acetaldehyde, a metabolite of alcohol, can damage the foetus and that the babies of chronically alcoholic mothers have a much increased chance of being inadequately nourished in the uterus and hence of being small-for-dates at birth and failing to thrive after birth. In one American study[2] it was found that the children of alcoholic mothers suffered a 30 – 50 per cent chance of 'the fetal alcohol syndrome' and among these the majority gave evidence of prenatal and postnatal growth deficiency, were delayed in their development, or were mentally defective. The authors suggest that although these babies suffered severe effects from alcohol there may be also a large number of babies of mothers who drink heavily but are not actually alcoholics, who show mild degrees of mental or growth retardation.

[1] *Federal Register* **43**, 114, 13 June (1978). US Department of Health, Education and Welfare.
[2] J.W. Hanson *et al.*; Fetal alcohol syndrome: experience with 41 patients, *Journal of the American Medical Association* **235**, 1458 – 60 (1976).

Birth at home

It is perplexing that some pregnant women can drink excessively and yet bear undamaged babies, whereas others drink relatively little and have babies who show the foetal alcohol syndrome. It has now been discovered that some women cannot safely drink at all during pregnancy and even a little alcohol will result in stunted growth and mental development. A Hungarian study[1] revealed that in women who are unable to metabolize acetaldehyde the foetal alcohol syndrome cannot be prevented by setting an upper limit to the daily alcohol consumption. It should be possible to screen women to discover their blood acetaldehyde level after drinking alcohol; then, when it surpasses a critical level, the woman can be advised to take no alcohol whatsoever during pregnancy.

In evidence to a United States Congress Committee on Health and the Environment (June 1978) a representative of the Proprietary Association of Drug Firms disclosed that research shows that 75 per cent of all illnesses were treated at first by self-medication with over-the-counter drugs. Another American study[2] examined the medicines taken by women during pregnancy and discovered that each woman took an average of 4.5 different drug preparations during her pregnancy. 8 out of 10 of these were taken without the doctor knowing. The other 2 were prescribed. They included aspirins, antacids, diuretics, cathartics, antibiotics, antihistamines, and barbiturates.

The placenta used to be thought of as a 'barrier'. It is, in fact, more like a sieve. When it starts to function at about the fifth week after conception, foreign substances diffuse passively across it to establish an equilibrium between the maternal and foetal bloodstreams. The rate at which this occurs is largely dependant on the concentration gradient, determined by the size, shape, and electrostatic charge of the molecules. If the molecules of the substance are of low weight (under 60) they can quickly cross the placenta, but large ones (over 1000) do so less readily. In substances with large molecules lipid solubility seems to be a more important factor in whether they cross the placenta in large quantities.[3]

Whether a drug affects the baby depends on (1) its toxicity,

[1] W. A. Bleyer *et al.*; Studies on the detection of adverse drug reaction in the newborn,*Journal of the American Medical Association* **213**, 12 (1970).

[2] Personal communication from Dr Peter Dunn, Reader in Perinatal Medicine, University of Bristol.

[3] *Drugs adversely affecting the human fetus.* Ross Laboratories, Columbus, Ohio (1971).

Drugs and diet in pregnancy

(2) the dose, (3) the stage of development the foetus has reached, (4) the susceptibility of the foetus, (5) predisposing conditions in the mother, and (6) whether the drug has widespread or very limited effects.[1] Probably not more than 2—3 per cent of developmental defects in human beings are due to drugs.[2]

Animal experiments cannot tell us with certainty whether pharmacological substances are teratogenic (damaging to the foetus) in human beings. Thalidomide, for example, was harmful in rabbits and monkeys but did not affect rats.

The baby is especially susceptible to the effects of teratogens in the first 12 weeks of pregnancy, during the period of organogenesis, when the main organs of the body are formed. It is particularly vulnerable before the mother is even certain that she is pregnant. Teratogenic effects have been reported from 11 days after conception. Up till the time when the placenta starts to function teratogens usually kill the foetus, which is then spontaneously aborted.

The nervous system is most likely to be affected by teratogens from the 15th to the 25th day after conception, the eyes from the 24th to the 40th day, the heart from the 20th to the 40th day, and the legs from the 24th to the 36th day.[3] After the first three months of pregnancy malformations as the result of drugs taken by the mother probably do not occur.

Teratogenic substances may affect the metabolism of the placenta on which the baby depends for its oxygenation and nutrition and for getting rid of waste products at any stage of pregnancy. This is why it is important to avoid all drugs unless they are essential for the mother's health.

In 1950 – 2 at the University of Chicago a study was done of DES (diethylstilboestrol), a synthetic hormone used to prevent miscarriage. It revealed a high incidence of breast cancer in those women who were given the drug. In 1971 further studies linked DES with a rare vaginal cancer or abnormal cell changes in the daughters of women who had the drug during pregnancy and

---

[1] Roger W. Hoag: Perinatal pharmacology, *Birth and the Family Journal,* **113** (1974).

[2] J. G. Wilson: Present status of drugs as teratogens in Man, *Teratology* **7**, 3 – 16 (1974).

[3] *Drugs adversely affecting the human fetus,* op. cit., referring to material in B. Mirkin, *Postgraduate Medicine* **47**, 91 (1970).

genital damage and infertility in their sons. The Federal Drug Administration withdrew approval of DES for use in preventing miscarriages, but it continued to be used as a feed additive to stimulate the growth of cattle, and since the hormone was still on the market (for the treatment of breast cancer, prostate cancer, and senile vaginitis) doctors could not be prevented from giving it to their patients. An FDA official, commenting in 1977, said, 'Unfortunately, some of the doctors out there are still prescribing that stuff.'[1] The most sound advice for any woman who thinks she may be having a miscarriage is to go to bed and rest until the bleeding has stopped or a miscarriage takes place.

Smallpox and rubella vaccination should not be done during pregnancy as they may have teratogenic effects.

In the United States diuretics are widely used by obstetricians to reduce fluid retention in pregnancy. Some pregnant women ask their doctors for diuretics to improve their appearance when they have mild oedema of the legs during hot weather. A certain degree of water retention is normal in pregnancy, and although swelling of hands and/or face should be treated as a warning signal that the blood pressure should be measured and that more rest and a better diet may be required, mild swelling of the legs and feet in very hot weather is normal. Ammonium chloride, the drug often used to treat the condition, tends to reduce the plasma volume,[2] and as a result the baby's blood pH, to below normal levels.

Hydralazine is a widely used drug to bring down blood pressure (anti-hypertensive). The mother may experience headaches, palpitations and hot flushes, and her heart may beat faster. The drug may slow down the flow of blood through the placenta, but as long as the effects on the placental circulation are watched carefully and it is not allowed to fall much below normal, effects on the baby are minimal.[3] Diazoxide, although it, too, can produce alarming results in the mother, increase in heart rate, headache, giddiness, hot flushes, nausea, and vomiting and water retention, also appears to have minimal effects on the baby.[4]

Magnesium sulphate is used to prevent convulsions in the mother

---

[1] Report in *New York Herald Tribune,* 14 December 1977.
[2] J. V. Kelly, Drugs used in the management of toxaemia of pregnancy, *Clinical Obstetrics, Gynecology* **20**, 395 – 410 (1977).
[3,4] Kelly, op. cit.

Drugs and diet in pregnancy

who has pre-eclampsia. Some studies have reported respiratory depression in babies of mothers who have had this drug.[1] Magnesium sulphate has been used for more than 50 years, however, and its effects on the baby are usually considered negligible as compared with the advantage to the mother who is suffering from toxaemia.

Valium (Diazepam) is widely used when the mother has toxaemia. It brings down her blood pressure effectively, but it passes rapidly to the foetus and levels in the foetus are higher than in the mother. The foetus can metabolize it only slowly, so after delivery the baby may be slow to suck. This drug can also result in a drop in the newborn's temperature and a slowing down of breathing.[2] Valium is used routinely as an effective tranquilizer and is offered in labour in some hospitals to any mother who appears anxious, fearful, or resistant to hospital policies.

Mild tranquillizers (the benzodiazepines) are sometimes prescribed in pregnancy and, when they are, their advantages probably outweigh any risks to the foetus. Sometimes, however, a woman takes stronger tranquillizers (the phenothiazines such as chlorpromazine and butyrophenones such as haloperidol) prescribed before she became pregnant. They are best avoided in pregnancy because of their possible effect on the baby's central and autonomic nervous systems. Chlorpromazine taken over a long period can cause damage to the foetal retina. Tranquillizers can sometimes also provoke allergic conditions.[3]

Lithium, used for the treatment of severe depression, can cause goitre in the foetus and is associated with nasal stuffiness, sleepiness, and feeding difficulties in the newborn. When a mother needs drug treatment of this kind the risk of affecting the baby is worth taking, but it should be remembered that drugging the baby may create further difficulties for the mother and make interaction with her baby harder than ever. This may increase rather than diminish her depression.

Aspirin (salicylates) used heavily in the last weeks of pregnancy can lead to short-term difficulties in blood-clotting, jaundice, and occasionally to damage to the central nervous system in the

---

[1] Kelly, op. cit.
[2] *Drugs adversely affecting the human fetus*, op. cit.

newborn baby. In a study of 272 deliveries 10 per cent of all
newborn babies were discovered to have salicylates in their cord
blood and some had concentrations above the usual analgesic levels
for adults.[1] A headache is best treated by rest in a quiet, darkened
room and, if possible, sleep.

Barbiturates are effective sedatives and are sometimes prescribed
in pregnancy, especially if the mother has toxaemia. Small oral
doses have least effect on the foetus, but large doses are likely to
cause respiratory depression in the newborn baby. Only those
sleeping pills which have been prescribed by the obstetrician should
be taken in pregnancy, and a milky drink, a boring book, and a
repertoire of relaxation exercises[2] is much better.

General anaesthetics should be avoided if possible during
pregnancy, although sometimes their use is unavoidable. If a
woman needs a tooth extracted she should tell her dentist she is

Among antibiotics the long-acting sulphonamides (used for the
treatment of urinary infections) should be avoided in the last weeks
of pregnancy, since they can result in jaundice and damage to the
central nervous system in the newborn.[3] Streptomycin taken
throughout pregnancy can affect the baby's hearing and may be
associated with skeletal damage. Tetracycline taken over a
prolonged period in late pregnancy can cause yellow staining of the
milk teeth with defects in the enamel.

Anticoagulants are sometimes prescribed in pregnancy. Warfarin
can affect the foetus at whatever stage of pregnancy it is taken.
Dicoumarol crosses the placenta freely and can cause neonatal
death. Heparin should be used when labour is imminent instead.
Small doses of vitamin K will quickly reverse the effects of
Dicoumarol.[4]

Women addicted to narcotic drugs, morphine and heroin, are
likely to give birth to babies who are already addicted in the uterus.
These babies suffer withdrawal symptoms which begin 1 – 3 days
following delivery, need to be protected from injuring themselves

[1] P. A. Palmisano and G. Cassady; Salicylate exposure in the perinate, *Journal of the American Medical Association,* 209 – 556 (1969).
[2] See Sheila Kitzinger: *The experience of childbirth,* op. cit., and *Journey through birth,* cassette tapes available through the National Childbirth Trust, 9 Queensborough Terrace, London, W2.
[3] Kelly, op. cit.
[4] Hoag, *Drugs adversely affecting the human fetus,* op. cit.

Drugs and diet in pregnancy

because they are irritable and twitching, have a characteristic high-pitched cry, and may suffer convulsions. I have seen these babies experiencing this terrible introduction to life in a large New York hospital. Approximately 1 in 3 of them die.

LSD (lysergic acid diethylamide) can produce chromosomal damage if taken in the first 3 months and can result in stunted growth in the baby.

In antenatal clinics, especially those attached to teaching hospitals, research is often undertaken into drugs. These have usually been very well tested on experimental animals first and will be prescribed in the hope that they have better effects than other drugs previously used to treat the condition from which the woman is suffering, hyperemesis (continual vomiting), urinary infection, high blood-pressure, etc. A pregnant woman has a right to know if she is part of a research series and to be fully informed about the likely effects and possible short- and long-term side effects of any drug or treatment used. The International Childbirth Education Association has prepared a Pregnant Patient's Bill of Rights and Responsibilities, part of which states:

The Pregnant Patient has the right, prior to the administration of any drug or procedure, to be informed by the health professional caring for her of any potential direct or indirect effect, risks or hazards to herself or her unborn or newborn infant which may result from the use of the drug or procedure prescribed for or administered to her during pregnancy, labor, birth or lactation.

The statement goes on to say that the woman has the right to determine for herself, without pressure from her attendant, whether she will accept the risks inherent in the proposed therapy or refuse a drug or procedure.

Although the woman having her baby at home usually knows her GP well and can discuss care with him or her, she may be having shared care between her GP and the Consultant Unit during her pregnancy. She owes it to her baby not to be passive about any proposed drugs or treatments which are advised but to ask questions, inform herself fully, and take active responsibility for her own and the baby's health.

This section has not been easy to write. No one wants to alarm expectant mothers unnecessarily. On the other hand it is doubtful whether the idea that the pregnant woman must be kept tranquil at all costs, and should rely on doctors to do what is best for her and her baby, is any longer valid (if it ever was) in the world of today. Part of taking responsibility for oneself and for the life of a new human being is discovering the facts, even when they are not pleasant, and weighing up the consequences of different kinds of action. To learn about the teratogenic effect of many pharmacological substances taken in pregnancy does not mean that a pregnant woman should refuse to take any medication. It does mean that a balance must be found between the possible risks to the foetus and the benefits to the mother and that no drugs, even aspirins or an occasional cigarette, should be taken without consideration of their effect on the baby.

Life styles

Draw up the dew. Swell with pacific violence.
Take shape in silence. Grow as the clouds grew.
Beautiful brood the cornlands, and you are heavy...[1]

Women give birth to healthy babies all over the world living under widely varied conditions, eating different kinds of foods, engaged in wide-ranging kinds of activity, living in inaccessible mountain villages, deep valleys and gorges, tundra, desert, frozen plains, jungles, on farms or in blocks of flats, in small towns and big cities. There is no one 'right' way to live during pregnancy, only a great many different ways. A pregnant woman has to work out for herself what kind of life style keeps her healthiest given the place where she lives, the kind of work she does, the diet to which she is accustomed, the exercise she enjoys, and her responsibilities to others in the family.

Obstetricians treat pathological conditions, seeking to eliminate the symptoms, but they are often powerless to affect the cause. There is no real cure for toxaemia of pregnancy (pre-eclampsia) for example. All the hospital can do is to provide bedrest, sedating drugs, and drugs to reduce the blood pressure and, once the baby appears to be safer out than in, to induce labour before term. Perhaps the seeds of toxaemia and hypertension are to be found in pregnant women's lifestyles which in a largely urban society are ill-adapted to pregnancy; their hectic, rushed lives, their often grossly

[1] C. Day Lewis from *Feathers to Iron,* The Hogarth Press (1936)

inadequate diets which may be high in calories but low in everything else, and the emotional stresses to which they are subject. The woman wanting to have her baby at home should adopt a lifestyle which makes the development of pre-eclamptic toxaemia unlikely. If she does develop the symptoms of toxaemia she will be advised to have her baby in hospital.

It is in fact not difficult to work out in early or mid-pregnancy whether or not your blood pressure is likely to shoot up in late pregnancy. (The time when it does so most often is in the last couple of weeks.) Norman Grant, Professor of Obstetrics at the University of Texas, checks the blood pressure with a woman lying on her left side and then asks her to roll over onto her back and takes it again.[1] If she is predisposed to hypertension the pressure shows a rise of 20 milliunits or more within one minute. 9 out of 10 women whose blood pressure does not rise under these conditions do not develop toxaemia, while three-quarters of those who have a positive 'roll-over' response get toxaemia, sometimes as much as 3 months later. It is probably worth asking your doctor at the antenatal clinic whether it is possible to have this simple routine test. If blood pressure is raised with the roll-over, preventive measures through rest and improved nutrition can then be taken.

In a discussion of the causes of hypertension in the general public (not pregnant women) two doctors at Charing Cross Hospital, London,[2] said that two major problems face us today..

The first is the extent to which hypertension and its related cardiovascular disorders are the outcome of a morbid relationship between the individual and his environment—that is, of a relationship that creates excessively severe and prolonged arousal leading to fatigue and exhaustion. The second is the extent to which relief from these disorders should be obtained by modifying the morbid relationships as opposed to treating the raised blood pressure pharmacologically as if it were a disease in its own right.

They went on to speak about 'maladaptive' behaviour which led to the admission of patients to hospital for the treatment of hypertension which they diagnosed as the cause of ill health in one-third of their hypertensive patients, and 'extreme frustration and

[1] Reported in *Newsweek,* 31 January 1977.
[2] P.G. F. Nixon and David H. Dighton: Meditation or Methyldopa? *British Medical Journal* **ii**, 525, 28 August 1976.

anger or despair and hopelessness' which they believed was responsible for the hypertension in two-thirds of their cases.

It is no denial of the stress of pregnancy on the whole maternal organism to ask whether the aetiology of toxaemia may not also derive in no small degree from maladaptive behaviour, and to suggest that anxiety, fatigue, inability to relax, and the loss of sleep that stems from these emotional states, may all contribute to a level of arousal which pushes the blood pressure up and results in pre-eclampsia.

Part of the treatment used by Nixon and Dighton was relaxation, transcendental meditation, or yoga and 'an attempt was made to teach every patient to recognize the level of arousal and fatigue that made his blood pressure high and to be responsible for his own care'.[1]

It is common practice for expectant mothers in my own childbirth education classes, on finding that their blood pressure is high at the antenatal clinic, to ask if they may have time to relax for 15 – 20 mintues and then to have it checked again. Most women are able to bring it down appreciably.

Learning how to recognize the signals from one's body that rest, a break in activities, exercise, or sleep is needed now can be a valuable bonus of childbirth education classes which is useful in the non-pregnant state too. But understanding how to relax can do more than that; it can be used to control systems in the body, to reduce the blood pressure, slow the heartbeat, and even to warm or cool down parts of the body. This is what is done when *biofeedback* machines are used, but if a woman has someone who can test her relaxation she may be able to achieve these results without expensive equipment. The lifting and letting drop of a wrist or elbow, ankle or knee by a partner is, in a sense, a biofeedback mechanism which can record resistance and tension. Once the woman has learned the different sensations of relaxation and tension (and these should be learned first), she herself knows immediately the helper begins to take the weight of a limb in his hand whether or not there is any resistance and soon becomes aware of residual tension in parts of the body she had previously thought relaxed. She often says, 'That arm isn't perfectly relaxed. It's up by my shoulder that it still feels a bit stiff', 'I haven't quite

[1] Nixon and Dighton, op. cit.

got that muscle released', 'There's a bit of tightness there still. Let's do it again.'

She also becomes aware of the rate and depth of breathing, which she can consciously control to attain better relaxation by letting it get slower and relaxing more and more with each long breath out, and of her heart rate, which, especially if she was excited, anxious, or rushed before starting to practice, she can observe changing to a slower rate.

Understanding relaxation also means that it is not restricted to a half-hour's or even an hour's practice a day but is incorporated into daily life. *Deep* relaxation practised regularly needs to be linked with *differential* relaxation in posture and movement. This is the art of using only those muscles which need to be used for any task or to maintain balance.

This reduces fatigue because energy is applied more rationally, and avoids the accumulation of residual tensions which contribute to the general static contraction of musculature when the body is held taut, ready for fight or flight, as it meets the stresses and threats of everyday life.

The study of relaxation can thus effect a re-ordering of the individual with her environment, and because the relaxed person sends out very different social signs from one who is tense, it may also change that environment. The adolescent who lunges heavily into the room, shoulders tense, jaw stiff, feet flung on the floor at each step, door banged behind her is telling everyone that she is 'fed up' or spoiling for a fight. The man who comes in from a dreadful day at the office with fists clenched, brow furrowed, smile glazed and still, back rigid as a ruler, shoulders bearing the weight of his burden, tells his wife, in effect, that he is not going to find it easy to enjoy an evening with her and probably will not be able to taste dinner, he is so preoccupied with worrying thoughts. The body is a messenger more powerful than language.

Thus relaxation can modify a morbid relationship with the environment and, because it changes physical behaviour and the expression of the body in posture, movement, gesture, and facial appearance, can also modify the social environment directly by having a positive effect on relationships both within and outside the family.

Pre-eclamptic toxaemia and other evidence of failure of the metabolism of the pregnant woman to adjust to the stresses confronting her is also frequently associated with a poor diet. In the past adequate diet has often been considered relatively unimportant in the pregnant woman because there was evidence that babies achieved good birth weights even when the mother was malnourished. Babies born in the Netherlands during the German occupation, when many mothers were suffering extreme hunger and diets low in both protein and calories, were only slightly below normal weights (although there were many more miscarriages, stillbirths, and babies who died shortly after birth). Studies now being done, however, are revealing that severe weight control in pregnancy may be hazardous for both mother and baby.

Since one of the earliest signs of toxaemia is sudden weight gain some obstetricians put the pregnant woman on a strict diet with reduced salt intake (which also has the effect of making many foods unpalatable), when there is evidence of considerable gains in the last three months of pregnancy. Some expectant mothers hope that by limiting food in pregnancy they will recover their figures more easily and so go on slimming diets of 1500 calories per day or less during pregnancy. These practices can be extremely dangerous for both the mother and her baby.[1]

Yet many women with perfectly normal pregnancies who go on to deliver healthy babies have what obstetricians see as an 'excessive weight gain'. Women with toxaemia tend to put on a lot of weight but this is probably a consequence rather than a cause of the toxaemia. There is no evidence that being on any type of diet or taking any kind of pills to reduce weight gain during pregnancy is as good as spontaneously keeping weight gain at about the right amount. It is important to note, too, that puffiness and swelling resulting from water retention is not by itself a pathological symptom and that to some degree it is 'a necessary and normal physiologic adaptation to pregnancy'[2] Studies in Sweden and elsewhere reveal that the woman who is slightly oedematous is *more* likely to have a straightforward labour and produce a healthy baby than the mother who has no water retention at all. 'Salt and edema are not the formidable enemies they are generally believed to be. On the contrary, they may be indispensable to the normal course of pregnancy.'[2]

[1] Gary K. Oakes and Ronald A. Chez: Nutrition in pregnancy. *Contemporary Obstetrics and Gynecology* **4**, 147 – 50 (1974).
[2] Volkaer, op. cit.

Drugs and diet in pregnancy

A good mixed diet, high in protein, vitamins, and minerals, with fresh fruit and vegetables or a salad at every meal, and restricted carbohydrates, seems sensible given our present state of knowledge. Obesity is associated with more obstetric difficulties and with medical problems such as hypertension, cardiac disease, and diabetes, all problems that can complicate the pregnancy and make hospital delivery necessary. It is important in the last three months of pregnancy to eat as the appetite dictates. If good eating habits have been learned before pregnancy started or in early pregnancy and 'junk foods' (fizzy drinks, packet puddings, and other prepared products which are often high in carbohydrates but low in any other food values) eliminated entirely from the diet, a woman can trust her own appetite to supply good nutrition for herself and her baby.

There is no reason why a woman should not have any particular food she fancies and it may well be that if she has a passionate desire for oranges or porridge or for any other similar food, this is an indication that such a food can provide something that is lacking in her diet. The well-known cravings of early pregnancy, enshrined and often exaggerated in popular myth, are often associated with nutritional inadequacies. Earth eating, well known among the poor in the southern states of the USA, has been clearly linked with iron deficiency, and the same association exists between low haemoglobin and a craving to chew ice. The woman who has bizarre cravings of this kind should carefully examine her diet to ensure that she has iron-rich foods. Some women report a craving for pickled foods and other substances high in salt in early pregnancy. This may be one indication of the increased need for salt in normal pregnancy. But when a woman wants large quantities of any food the consumption of which is likely to lead to an unbalanced diet, she should remember that her unborn baby depends on her for adequate nutrition in the uterus.

There are two periods of rapid development of brain cells in the foetus, the first occurring at 20 weeks and the second at 36 weeks, at which times the brain may be most vulnerable to maternal malnutrition. Attempts to avoid excessive weight gain by strict dieting in late pregnancy, or cutting out salt, an increased need for which is a normal accompaniment of pregnancy, just when the foetus is approaching its final growth spurt, impairs the baby's growth after birth as well as producing a newborn who

95

has been deprived of nutrition in the uterus.[1]

Tom Brewer has drawn attention to the way in which the drug industry in the United States, having put oral thiazide diuretics on the market in the late 1950s, 'aggressively promoted not only these diuretic pills but also their own low-salt, low-calorie diet sheets', which he calls 'a pernicious error which laid the groundwork for middle-class pregnancy malnutrition on an unprecedented scale'.[2] He asserts that doctors give only 'symptomatic treatment of the results of social and economic neglect'.[3]

The poor and undernourished have always had more 'reproductive casualties', including more premature labours, more undersize babies and babies suffering from the respiratory distress syndrome, more obstetric difficulties, more stillbirths and deaths in the first week of life and more spastic and mentally retarded babies. Epilepsy is ten times more common in the United States among those at the bottom of the socio-economic scale than in those at the top. Brewer points out that this has sometimes been explained by genetic inferiority and 'then there is nothing anyone in authority can do except perhaps build more institutions to care for the retarded'.[4] He has shown how giving these pregnant women adequate nutrition enables them to bear heavier, healthier babies.

Studies show that malnutrition is not confined to the poor. The 1968 – 70 Ten State Nutrition Survey in the USA disclosed that 'iron-deficiency anaemia, protein-calorie malnutrition, delayed growth and development, gross obesity, scurvy, rickets and beri-beri were widespread among the poor *and the non-poor,* among Black, White and Spanish Americans',[5] Low-calorie diets with diuretics increase this pre-existing malnutrition among pregnant women.

The vegetarian expectant mother

In reviewing her daily diet, the vegetarian who is planning to have

[1] I. Blumenthal: Diet and diuretics in pregnancy and subsequent growth of offspring. *British Medical Journal* ii, 753 (1976).

[2] Food, salt, water and pregnancy, *Keeping Abreast Journal* **2,** (4) (1977).

[3] Personal communication.

[4] Gail Sforza Brewer and Tom Brewer: *What every pregnant woman should know.* Random House, New York (1977).

[5] Barbara Luke: A nutritional assessment of the expectant mother, *Keeping Abreast Journal* **2** (4) (1977).

her baby at home should make certain that she is having adequate protein in the form of milk, cheese and eggs, or plant proteins (beans, nuts, seeds and grains). Roughly speaking the lacto-vegetarian needs 3-4 servings of milk or milk products each day, complemented by plant foods, grain products, a dark green vegetable and a fruit or vegetable especially rich in vitamin C. Most lacto-vegetarians have this anyway.

The woman who does not eat fish or vegetables grown in iodine-rich soil should have iodized salt. The iodine-deficient mother may bear a mentally handicapped baby. For years I thought that sea-salt contained iodine. It does not. Buy iodized salt and if the family likes the strong taste of sea-salt mix the two together.

The Vegan or woman on one of the 10 different macrobiotic diets needs to be more careful. Severe nutritional deficiencies result from diets of brown rice alone and marked restriction of fluids.[1,2,3] The pregnant woman should drink freely. 3 quarts of fluids a day are not too much and help to avoid constipation and keep the kidneys working well.

The people of the Farm, Tennessee, are quite frank that when they first moved from California to Tennessee they suffered nutritional inadequacies which affected childbearing until they obtained dietary advice. Subsequently the nutritionist for the commune outlined a diet based on soybeans used in tortillas, burgers, soymilk, yoghurt, ice cream, soy curd cheese, tofu (Japanese bean curd), and texturized vegetable protein. She suggests taking about 30 per cent more protein and vitamins than before pregnancy, brewer's yeast because of its B vitamins, and plenty of vegetables to ensure cellulose to prevent constipation, dark green vegetables because of their high vitamin C and A content, and folic acid. The need for folic acid doubles during pregnancy. Lack of it is associated with accidental bleeding and haemorrhage. Many obstetricians prescribe folic acid supplements. Vegans and those on macrobiotic diets get no vitamin B_{12} unless they take yeast or tex-

[1] Eleanor R. Williams: Nutrition: vegetarian diets in pregnancy. *Birth and the Family Journal* 3, 2 (1976).

[2] Committee on Nutritional Misinformation, Food and Nutrition Board, National Research Council: Vegetarian diets. *Journal of American Dietet. Association* 65, 121-2 (1974).

[3] Darla Erhard: The new vegetarians: the Zen macrobiotic movement and the other cults based on vegetarianism. *Nutrition Today* 9, 20 – 5 (1974).

turized vegetable proteins. This must be taken regularly as it is only absorbed in small quantities. A tablet containing 10 mg of vitamin B_{12} every day is a sensible addition to the diet of a vegetarian who eats no animal products. Vitamin B_{12} deficiency can lead to degeneration of the spinal cord and megablastic anaemia.

Protein can be obtained from a daily large cup of soybeans and a pint of soymilk or yoghurt. The Farm also recommends soybean-based snacks during pregnancy such as soynuts or peanut butter on celery or biscuits. Soybeans contain only one-fifth of the amount of calcium in cow's milk. A calcium supplement may also be advisable—1 gram a day as two 500-mg or three 5-grain tablets. The calcification of the foetal bones takes place in the last part of pregnancy.

The vegetarian who eats no animal products should learn how to balance the amino acids in different kinds of plant proteins so that all the eight essential amino acids are obtained each day. The body is able then to synthesize its own protein. This can be learned from *Diet for a small planet* by Frances M. Lappé, Ballantine Books, New York (1975) and *Recipes for a small planet* by Ellen B. Ewald, Ballantine Books, New York (1973). For example, a mixture of oats, wheat germ, sesame seeds, sunflower seeds, walnuts, raisins, a little oil, and some honey taken with soymilk for breakfast is a combination of foods that provides complementary amino acids.[1] Salted peanuts together with some soymilk do for a snack. Spanish soybeans, one of the recipes in *Recipes for a small planet,* over rice and bulgur wheat together with a salad can be followed by soybean yoghurt with fruit.

Blood tests in pregnancy will indicate whether the haemoglobin level is low and the obstetrician may prescribe extra iron. Severely anaemic mothers are more likely to have premature and stillborn babies,[2] and to suffer exhaustion and depression post-partum. The World Health Organization recommends iron supplements for all pregnant women since it is difficult to obtain adequate iron from many kinds of diet, but if you are having a good diet these should be unnecessary. It is probably wise to delay starting iron until after the first three months of pregnancy anyway, as it makes some women feel nauseous.

[1] Eleanor R. Williams, op. cit.
[2] E. F. Patrice Jelliffe: Effect of maternal dietary on fetal and subsequent child health and development. *Keeping Abreast Journal* 2 (4) (1977).

Drugs and diet in pregnancy

The drugs we choose to introduce into our blood streams in pregnancy, the food we eat, the state of contraction we allow our muscles to remain in, the anxieties by which we let ourselves be gripped, can all affect the baby whose life is unfolding in the depths of a woman's body. Every pregnant woman owes it to herself and to her unborn child to offer to her baby her body at its healthiest.

7

The other child

WOMEN expecting a second baby are often deeply concerned that the separation from a toddler involved in a hospital birth will prove disturbing for the older child. The occasion on which a new member is introduced into the family, one who is a potential rival to the ex-baby, seems to be the least suitable time for the mother to leave home.

They also want to make the birth of the baby not only frictionless but a joy for the older one too and to create the atmosphere in which it is a truly family event. This is one strong reason why a mother may consider having a birth at home.

Some hospitals, as we have seen already, do not allow visiting by other children except at very restricted times. Most do not permit them to be present at all during labour. At the time of writing no British hospitals allow them at delivery; and in some the older child is never even allowed to hold the baby. This is hard on the displaced baby who must surrender his or her unique place as the youngest or the only child in the family at the same time that there is traumatic separation from the mother and the excitement of a crisis in which everyone is involved. It does not help at all to present the new baby as a gift for the older child somehow mysteriously produced by the hospital, one which apparently injures the mother so that she must lie in bed in a large and frightening place where ill people go, surrounded by crisply efficient nurses and imposing doctors in white coats.

In hospital the baby may be in a plastic box in a nursery with a great many other babies and can only be glimpsed through glass or at the end of the mother's bed where the older child is supposed to admire it but not touch. The new baby is the centre of attention and the older child is just an onlooker in a strange building. Many hospitals have rules which prevent the child climbing on or in to the mother's bed for a cuddle. The mother is turned into a 'patient', a person towards whom the child must behave in a different way.

Birth at home

The only thing he or she can do is to select or make a present for the mother to take to hospital. When I was compiling my study of British maternity hospitals[1] there was an account from a woman whose little girl had brought her a box of multicoloured tissues. The mother put them on her locker so that when the child came at visiting time she should see that the gift was being used. However the ward Sister insisted that all unnecessary, untidy objects on lockers were cleared before visiting, reprimanded the mother for her untidiness, and removed the box. The mother, who was a school teacher and used to being fairly authoritative and capable, was surprised at the way in which she allowed this to happen and explained it in terms of the vulnerability which patients in hospital feel and the special sensitivity of new mothers. There are obviously a great many wards in which such things do not happen, but that the hospital environment *ever* permits them to occur is a reason why some women seek an alternative setting for childbirth when there are no special high-risk factors for choosing hospital birth.

During delivery

Accounts of home births from women who already have children invariably stress the advantages for the older child and the positive effect on relationships in the family.[2].

My baby was born just as my three-year-old son awoke. Within half an hour of delivery he was sitting with his sister as she sucked at the breast.

Julie woke up to find a sister had been born during the night just as we had told her it would happen. We were the happiest little family in the world.

I was able to play with my little girl (during the late first stage of labour)—although I did have to draw the line when she wanted to bounce on my tummy! Suddenly I knew I was about to reach stage two—so I told Helen I was going upstairs to have our baby and she would be able to see it soon ... and that's what happened, 15 minutes of very satisfying pushing and I saw Diggory's head appear in the mirror that Mark held and then he was born... The baby was put to the breast and started to suck at once and he looked so content. ... Helen came in at this point and decided to help her brother by sucking at the other side! Great celebrations—arrival of

[1] *Good birth guide.* Fontana, London (1979).
[2] See Sheila Kitzinger: Women's experiences of birth at home. In *The place of birth* (ed. Sheila Kitzinger and John Davis). Oxford University Press (1978).

The other child

Toby (older child) from school—bottle of champagne—big cuddles all round. I've never felt happier in my life.

Another woman's daughters had been sitting in bed reading, waiting for the call which meant they were allowed in:

I was able to lift my baby onto my stomach, gently massaging his skin. The light was dim, the room and I warm (no hypothermia)—but I did forget to be quiet, and laughed and called the waiting older girls to come and pat their seconds-old brother. It meant a lot to them to hear him born. ... And a little later ... I had a delicious bath, while my husband, helped by our two girls, slowly bathed the baby beside me.[1]

Some mothers are anxious in advance in case an older child wakes up when they are in strong labour or wanders into the room as they are trying to cope with a difficult contraction. They wonder what the effect might be on the child of seeing blood or witnessing pain. Yet children seem to take these experiences in their stride, provided adults do. Children pick up adult attitudes and if they are embarrassed or anxious this is readily conveyed to the child even though no word is spoken. It is therefore very important from this point of view alone that husband and wife are agreed about the kind of birth they want and how they are going to create the right environment for it, that the husband is knowledgeable and prepared for being a birth assistant, and that he can give the child the assurance of normality.

The relationship of the parents with professional birth attendants is also important. The child must feel that his parents can cope and that any strangers involved are there because the parents want them to be there and are in partnership with them, rather than that those outside the family have taken over control and the parents are rendered powerless.

Some mothers believe it might be a valuable experience for an older child to be present at the birth. Children will quite naturally go in and out of their mother's room while labour is taking place if they understand what is happening, have seen her practising her breathing and relaxation and have become friendly with the midwife and family doctor in advance. Once contractions are coming every 2 or 3 minutes a woman may find it easier to concentrate without older children there. Only she will know and

[1] Rachel Davies: A sensitive approach to childbirth. *Nursing Times* 9 February 1978.

Birth at home

she should keep an open mind and act as she feels at the time. She can explain that she is 'working very hard' and has to 'think', 'make pictures' in her head, 'breathe with the tightenings', or whatever else the children will understand. A child can feel the work the uterus is doing by resting a hand on the fundus.

Alternative activity and alternative care for the older child should always be available in case the mother finds the child's presence distracting or the child wants to do something else. In fact, most children who are present during labour seem to accept it as natural. Any child soon realizes that mother and father are 'busy'. One of three years or so can help by wringing out a face cloth in iced water to mop his mother's brow or doing other simple tasks which make of the birth a family activity. Picture books and playthings can be provided in a corner of the room and some private territory created for the older child where he can go if he wishes.

Parents should discuss what it is they hope the experience of birth at home may mean for their other child and how the environment and their own words and actions can affect this. When I was interviewing Zulu folk midwives and witchdoctors about childbirth I learned that traditionally children are brought to witness birth as an important part of their education. It takes place in a room which has been specially cleaned and decorated with beautiful carvings and other objects because the first thing the newborn baby sees should be lovely. The mother is not in bed, but kneeling on the floor helped by other women. She is engaged in an active task for which she is given assistance by women whom the children already know well. Thus the social relationships of those present at birth and the physical environment are markedly different from that in which birth usually takes place in our Westen technological culture.

In our society too home birth makes it possible to provide an environment in which fantasies of injury and the association of birth with anguish and threat are not nourished, but on the contrary birth is witnessed as a miracle. All children probably wonder how babies get out of their mothers' bodies, and even when given accurate information wonder how they can pass through that tiny hole. A little girl realizes that it hurts to push anything hard into her vagina and during her mother's pregnancy may experiment with a thimble, button, doll's tea cup or other object because she is anxious about this. This is a way in which she is asking for further information; she is not convinced that the baby can emerge without injuring her mother. Parents should be ready to explain to both girls and boys that the inside of the vagina is soft and 'stretchy' so that it can open up when the baby is pressing down from above. If there is among the child's playthings a fan or concertina or anything which spreads out this can be demonstrated. Illustrations in the New York Maternity Center's *Birth Atlas* are excellent for this, too. An NCT[1] antenatal teacher may have a doll and 'baby box' with a foam rubber 'perineum' and can show the child what happens.

Children may also want to know the mechanics of uterine action. Explain that the uterus is a big muscle, 'like the muscle in your arm', and show how with a hand on the biceps the child can feel the muscle tighten and go hard and then relax and go soft. The uterus tightens like this but without the mother having to tell it to; 'it just happens, like your heart beating, when it is time for the baby to be born'. Other ideas for explaining the physiology of labour and delivery and the language in which they can be described, are contained in a book I wrote for childbirth educators, teachers, midwives, and others, *Education and counselling for childbirth*.[2] The photographs in *A child is born*[3] may be useful and the text can help parents talk about what is happening as the baby grows inside the uterus.

The older child may also go with mother and father to the antenatal clinic or GP's surgery and learn that the doctor and midwife are friends. When the foetal heart can be heard clearly the child can hear it through the stethoscope or better still by the sonic aid. Ideally this should happen whether the baby is to be born at home or in hospital, but in a busy hospital antenatal clinic staff may feel that they cannot cope with husbands, let alone other children. If you attend a large, rather impersonal clinic it may be worth speaking to the Sister and saying that you would like to have your next appointment at a time when this could be done.

There will be many opportunities as pregnancy progresses for the child to feel the baby kicking and to realize that there is not just an anonymous, nondescript 'thing' in there, but a person. It may be

[1] The National Childbirth Trust, 9 Queensborough Terrace, London W2.
[2] Bailliere Tindall, London (1977).
[3] Lennart Nielsen *et al.* Allen Lane, London (1978).

important for a child to understand that a baby is not passive, like a doll or teddy bear, but has vitality and urgent needs that must be met. Once the baby is born, it can be hard for a toddler to appreciate that these needs must sometimes be satisfied before his own requests for a piggyback ride or a game of hide and seek are met, and in so far as the child can be prepared in advance for this the way can be paved for postpartum adjustments in the family.

The older child can be helped to feel the different parts of the baby through the abdominal wall. Rest-time, when mother and child lie down together or any occasion when they are both relaxed, is good for this.

On the other hand parents should be warned of projecting onto the child, especially one of under four years, their own pleasure in the forthcoming birth and expecting him or her to have similar emotions. It is important to be observant and to remain open to the child's own feelings. As the mother becomes preoccupied with the life inside her and the baby's arrival the child may wonder whether he is still loved, and whether there will be enough love to 'go round' when the baby is born. Inevitably after the birth the older child has less of the mother's time and attention. The parents can discuss practical arrangements with the child and perhaps say, 'Oh dear, we're going to be busy!' and help the child see that although the baby is wanted it is not going to be entirely undiluted pleasure for anyone. When the parents express rather more negative emotions like this they in effect give the child 'permission' also to express negative feelings about the baby.

If a child is to be present at delivery it is especially important that he knows where the baby is coming from and how it is born, is used to seeing his mother's naked body and has seen her practising her relaxation and breathing for labour. The midwife will want to know that there is someone available to care for the older child and that it is not a question of him having to be in the room because there is nowhere else for him to go. Discuss how you feel about the child's presence with your midwife in advance and give them ample opportunity to get to know each other by inviting her round for a meal or other social occasion. This is where domiciliary antenatal visits are a great help and children get used to seeing the midwife coming in and examining the mother. One mother said of her midwife[1]:

[1] *The place of birth,* op. cit.

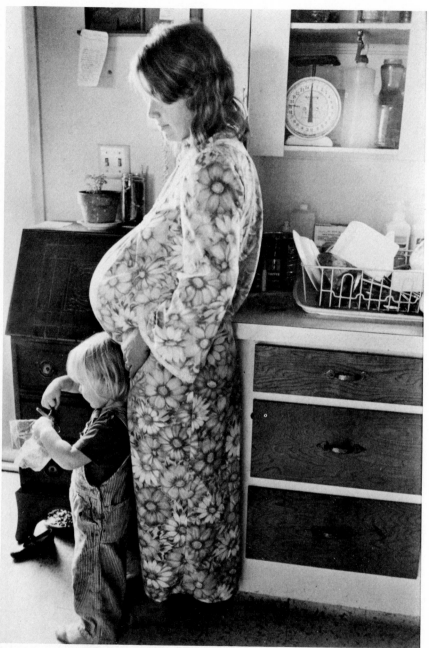

A woman in early labour, comfortable in an upright position and walking about, with her toddler. Continuing household activities and letting gravity help is one advantage of labouring at home.

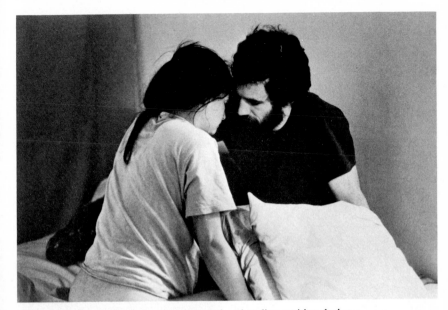

A couple on their bed together, the woman in a kneeling position during a
contraction, as her husband gives quiet encouragement. Attendants wait nearby,
giving them privacy.

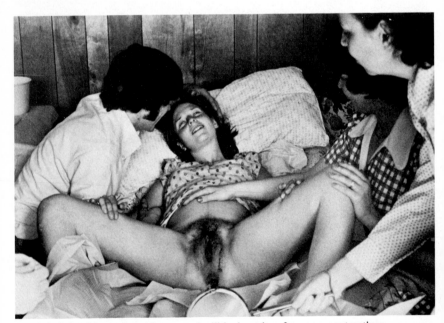

The baby's head is on the perineum and will be born in a few more contractions.
The woman's mother holds a mirror so she can catch the first glimpse of her
baby.

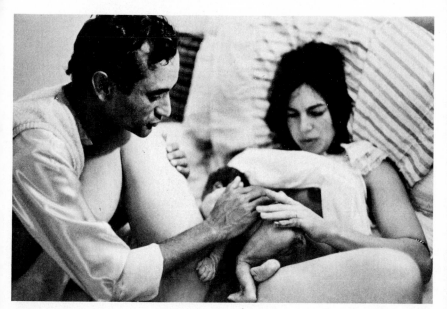

A mother lifts her baby up on to her abdomen and both parents stroke their newborn child, the cord still attached.

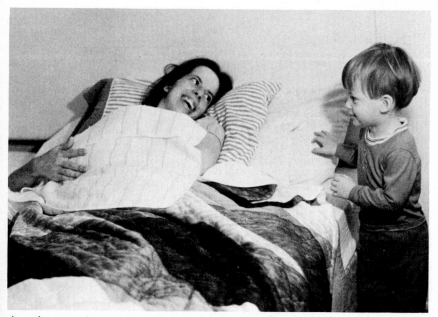

A mother greets her two year old who has woken up from his rest and come to see the new baby.

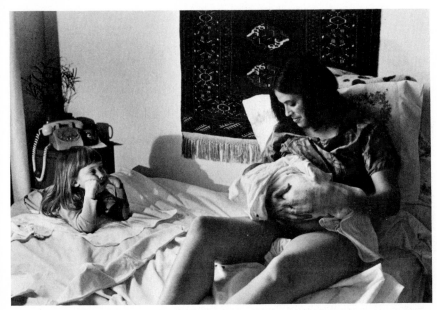

A four year old watches her mother and new sister shortly after delivery.

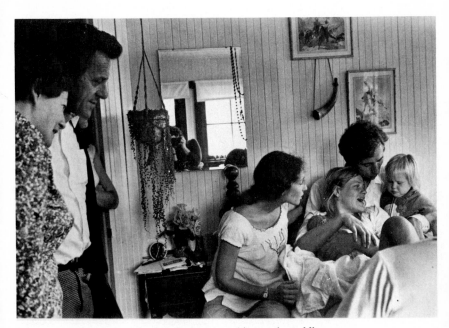

The new family together, the grandparents watching as the toddler seems overwhelmed by the intensity of her emotions just after birth.

The other child

She was wonderful. ... She visited me at home in the early stages of my pregnancy, and chatted as a friend would, over a cup of coffee. ... As my pregnancy progressed she called at the house once a week for her own personal check-up. She made friends with my three-year-old, letting her feel my tummy and listen to the baby's heartbeat. My doctor also always found time to explain things to my toddler.

Another mother wrote:

It was such a family affair. Emma and James had got to know the midwife well during the previous nine months and looked forward to her visits. They were able to come and see the baby about five minutes after he was born and in fact helped the midwife to bath and dress him. I'll never forget seeing them rushing backwards and forwards with soap, talc, hairbrush, etc.—they were so pleased that at last this much-talked-about baby was a reality.

After the delivery

Once the baby is born other children in the family can be involved immediately, can touch the baby and feel its tight hand-grip, if the temperature of the room is high enough can help in bathing it, and can help select clothes for and dress the baby. The mother's bed can become the centre of wonder.

When our fifth daughter was born early in the morning one of the four-year-old twins heard her birth cry and dashed up from the downstairs nursery. The things children remember about birth may not be those adults find the most significant, however. She remembers noticing that the furniture had been moved and that the bed was in a different place and thought this was very exciting, so she went to get her sisters. They all four trooped into the bedroom in new flower-sprigged nightdresses put ready for this special occasion as their father filmed them. The three-year-old had something in her hand and she uncurled the baby's fingers and slipped it into her fist; it was a tiny plastic doll which she must have thought would be about the right size for a new baby. One of the four-year-olds was interested in the placenta and how it worked. Everyone wanted to hold the baby, but first the cord needed trimming a little as my husband had cut it at some distance from the baby 'just in case'. Then they washed her as she lay on my lap and found her some clothes and together we dressed her. Inside the wardrobe was a baby doll for each girl. Jenny had been born quickly before we had had time to call the midwife, and it was only after this and we had all had a celebratory cup of tea together that I remembered to phone the midwife. She was *our* baby from the start.

One mother, commenting on the way in which the birth was 'always and exclusively ours as a family' and comparing it favourably with a previous hospital birth said:

> The midwife asked us every day how the baby was, and the children delighted in telling her all that had happened since her last visit. These may appear to be trivial details. But when I read of the break-up of families perhaps they are not so trivial, but vitally important factors instead.

Some parents hide away toys which they say are 'a present from the baby'. Although it is a good idea to mark the festivity of the occasion any child of two or older realizes that the new baby is incapable of giving presents. A doll, towards whom the child, whether girl or boy, can express all the ambivalent emotions he or she may be experiencing and can care for or reject at different times can provide parents with clues about the child's feelings. Some parents give a longed-for puppy, kitten, or other pet, but the child should be old enough to look after a living creature as it should be cared for.

When a new baby arrives the older child needs to be assured of his or her unique place in the family and in the parents' love. This can produce stress for the mother as she begins to learn about her baby and it is often a time when the older child regresses. He may need to go back into nappies or starts wetting the bed when he has not been doing so for some time; he demands to be spoonfed or suckled or to have a bottle, or gets finicky about food. He may not settle well at night and need a nightlight or insist on coming into the parents' bed. All this is normal. A strategy should be worked out in advance by the parents and they should decide together on their responses.

The convention by which birth announcements declare that Sarah is a sister for Andrew or Paul is a brother for Jane are misleading. The new baby is clearly not a present for the older child and a child who has been told it is may justifiably feel cheated. Adults watch carefully to see that no harm comes to the baby when the older child explores him and pokes around at his interesting looking eyes and mouth. The baby cannot join in games. It howls and wets and dirties nappies and no one seems to mind; and it latches on to the mother's breast as if it is going to eat her up.

Grandparents may offer to have an older child to stay with them when the new baby is due. This is probably not a good idea. How would you feel if you went away only to return home to discover that a complete stranger had taken your place and that your husband, whilst lying in bed cuddling the newcomer much of the day, was going on about how adorable she was, how he is sure you will love her and be a marvellous companion for her, and wouldn't you like to help look after her?

If older children enjoy staying with grandparents this can be arranged for a short time a few days after the birth. The initial excitement for the children has worn off by then. It allows them to participate in the events surrounding the birth and greet the new baby, while letting the parents have some time alone together a short time after.

No parent should believe that careful planning beforehand and sustained affection can completely eliminate the ex-baby's hostility towards the newborn child, although it may not be evident for some months following the birth. It is a normal part of the relationships between siblings and one which can enable them to learn to handle jealousy in adult life. The child who has never been anything but the centre of parental attention starts off emotionally as a handicapped adult. Rivalry often first becomes overt when the mobile and inquisitive baby towards the end of its first year knocks down laboriously built towers of bricks created by the older child, pulls a doll onto the floor and sucks its hair, or seizes the older child's cherished possession and does not surrender it until forced to do so. So it is especially at the end of the first and in the second year of life that the baby confronts the older child as an adversary in direct competition over playthings and possession of the mother. Parents should not be too sanguine about the child who successfully masks all hostility to the baby at this stage, for he may feel that it is too dangerous to express and will incur parental withdrawal of love. It is useful for a parent to be able to say, 'When my little brother was born I thought my Mummy loved the baby more than me', or 'When my younger sister spoiled my sandcastle I remember I felt *very* cross. I wanted to kill her!' Grandmothers and fathers can often tell children stories about when their mothers and fathers were children and some of these stories can illustrate and give adult assent to the reality and intensity of emotions felt in childhood and the manner in which they found expression, in a way which is remarkably satisfying for a small child. (The *My naughty little sister*[1] stories, which were very popular with our girls, are stories in this genre too.)

The father's role and his relationship with the older child is vitally important in the time following the birth of a new baby. Whenever possible he should take over tasks like helping the child to dress and undress, do up buttons, bath, settle down at night, and can spend time talking with him, go for walks, play games, or prepare a meal which they eat together while the mother is having a quiet meal in bed. This is not just a question of helping his wife but of fulfilling the child's emotional needs and giving *active fathering* at a time when change in the family can produce threatening insecurity for the displaced child. In the father's absence another woman may share this care of the child in return for help with her own child at another time. All this is happening, however, at a time when the older child at 2½ or so may be going through a 'clinging stage' and unless a good relationship has already been formed with the adult who helps it is too much to expect the child to co-operate with such plans, however good they seem to the adults concerned.

Grandparents often fill such a role admirably and may derive great joy from helping in this way. It is much more important for them to do this than to help with the new baby. The mother herself needs to learn about her baby and discover its rhythms. But in spending time with the older child grandparents can help create for the mother and baby a sanctuary in which they begin to know each other.

The older child must not feel ejected from this sanctuary. If 'Mummy is resting now' or 'Mummy is feeding the baby' ways must be found in which the toddler can cuddle up and share in the love. Unfortunately two and three-year olds tend to wriggle and resting together may only be tolerable in a very large bed in which the child can be nested down in pillows, separated from mother and baby by a bolster or pillows rather like Puritan lovers who 'bundled'.

When possible the mother can see to the toddler's requirements *before* dealing with the baby. With a little imagination the older child's wants can be foreseen. My oldest child found it difficult to

[1] Dorothy Edwards, Penguin, Harmondsworth (1969)

cope emotionally with newborn twin sisters when she was not yet two herself, and always wanted a drink of water when I was breast-feeding. So I planned on having a drink with her each time I picked up a baby to feed and made it ready first. In a cupboard in the bedroom toys were kept specially for feeding times and we often read a book together as I cuddled a baby in one arm and the older child in the other, or she sat in the middle of the big bed with one while I fed the other and we listened to some music or I read a story to her.

When a new baby comes the older child needs not only to be loved, but to be shown that she is loved, and this is most easily and satisfyingly achieved in the security of the home, when there is no separation from the mother and where birth is an integral part of the natural unfolding of family life. Birth at home is an opportunity for older children to see childbirth as a normal life crisis, to share in the joy of bringing into the world a new human being, to perceive something of the miracle of birth and, however young they are, to contribute to what should be a family occasion.

8

Labour
I: The father's role

IN many ways it can be more difficult for a man to feel himself a father than it is for a woman to feel herself a mother. The child is not born from his body. Women are often anxious that they will not be able to produce the appropriate maternal feelings after the baby is born. Men may have similar anxieties about the challenging transition to fatherhood, but are able to hide them in asserting a socially conventional 'masculine' identity outside the home, emphasizing their role as 'providers' and trusting that the woman will cope with the baby. When this happens the expectant mother who is already unsure of herself and her own capacity to mother becomes even more anxious; her husband is leaving it all to her. The couple having a baby at home realize that there is no solution in this division of emotional and parental responsibility. The man knows that he will be needed at the time of birth, that his wife depends on him and that he is bound to get deeply involved in everything that happens.

In hospital birth today the father is often able to help his wife, to remind her about her breathing and relaxation, rub her back, help her change position and be an onlooker at the birth, but as we have seen he is a member of a 'team' and from the staff's point of view the one most easily dispensed with at that; at the first sign of any difficulty or real work to be done he is likely to be sent out. He is allowed and sometimes even welcomed, but he is not *necessary*. Couples who have had a baby in hospital and then have had the next one at home comment on the very different role of the father in the home birth and the mother often says things like 'I couldn't have done it without him'. It obviously appears to many women incomprehensible that they could have had their babies without their partners there helping and supporting them, and other relationships, with the midwife and doctor for example, pale into insignificance beside the husband – wife relationship. The man feels himself a father even before the baby is delivered. The coming to birth of the child is an integral part of the birth of a man as a father.

A man can absent himself from the birth, which many men still consider the quintessence of dangerous and polluting female body functions. Judaeo-Christian society has traditionally emphasized complete separateness between male and female body functions. The agricultural societies of the past kept male and female roles distinct and differences in the knowledge held by men and women were also maintained. Even now in Mediterranean cultures male and female represent bipolar categories of human nature, men being intelligent, women stupid; men strong-minded, women credulous; men brave, women fearful; men reliable and women unreliable; men strong, women weak; men responsible and women irresponsible.[1,2]

The mystique of the female world and especially the dark and bloody secret of the female body is considered not only something which men can never know or understand but also as something which must be kept completely separate because the man contaminated by them can no longer be truly male. This is the powerful but often unspoken idea behind many men's avoidance of childbirth and their conviction that it is best to 'leave it to the professional'. It is why they have preferred to go to the pub to drink the labour through or to suffer agonies in a hospital waiting room smoking endless cigarettes rather than witness any of what is for them a tabooed female process.

There are still men today who prefer to know nothing about childbirth, who distrust their own emotional reactions, dread seeing their wives in pain while, as they say, they are 'not able to do anything about it', and who fear that participating in birth would somehow deprive them of their masculinity. But in a rapidly changing society, new concepts concerning the relationships between men and women and between parents and children, and the significance which is now being given to the home as 'a private refuge from increasing alienation' at work,[3] have brought with

---

[1] Juliet de Boulay: *Portrait of a Greek mountain village.* Oxford University Press, (1974).

[2] Sheila Kitzinger: *Women as mothers.* Fontana, London (1978).

[3] Joel Richman and W. O. Goldthorp: In *The place of birth;* op. cit.

them a fresh approach to the father's role in childbirth.

As we saw in Chapter 2, wanting the husband to be able to share fully in the birth and a conviction that this would happen most easily in his own home was one of the main reasons why many of the women whose home-birth accounts I studied chose home in the first place. They often did so because of previous unhappy hospital experiences, for in spite of policies about husbands being present in labour and at delivery the father is often treated as a 'peripheral appendage'[1] to the mother, his role in the delivery room is often afforded only token recognition as 'unpaid comforter alleviating staff shortages'[1] and he feels out of place in hospital.

At home, on familiar territory which he himself controls, the man is able to retain his own identity as a person and not just as the labouring woman's partner, in a way which it is often impossible for him to do in hospital. There is little point, for example, in a father being gowned and dressed in other sterile garments in his own home. The woman is giving birth in the bed which he has recently vacated and which he will often get back into again once the baby is delivered. He sits or lies on the bed beside her, an impossibiliity on the high, hard, and narrow hospital delivery table, and has close and spontaneous physical contact with his wife in a way which may be frowned on in the kind of hospital where fathers are seen as harbouring dangerous bacteria. In home birth the man takes on an active role and does so because his contribution is needed. No concessions need to be made so that he can be with his wife; he is simply there because she depends on him; the midwife, too, relies on his help and his knowledge of his wife and the surroundings. When the midwife asks for anything he knows where to find it. He offers to make a pot of tea and brings it up for them; he regulates the temperature of the room, moves any furniture that may be in the way. He is host as well as husband.

At home he shares with his wife in an intimate and private experience which is often in marked contrast to an event taking place in the public arena of the hospital delivery room, where there is not only a team of midwives and doctors but also students, people to whom he is never introduced and whose names he only catches by hearing them mentioned by other members of staff. Individuals come and go without warning. Not only do unknown

[1] Richman and Goldthorp, op. cit.

staff members enter to give messages but often just as one is getting used to a familiar figure he or she goes off duty to be replaced by somebody new. Women often say they find this 'unsettling' or 'confusing'. It is equally confusing for fathers.

For some couples wanting home birth is also part of a philosophy of life which puts emphasis on relationships between people in mutual dependence and caring, and they see qualities of individual caring submerged by bureaucratized systems of management and control in hospital childbirth. A man who believes this sees it as part of his responsibility to his wife and child actively to share in the birth and to help in creating an environment which is qualitatively different from that in most hospitals. One man, for example, said that he toured the labour suite of the local hospital,

and after that we were sure that we didn't want to have our child come into a group of strangers at such a place but rather with the loving circle of family and friends in a familiar setting. We also felt strongly that our child should emerge into her father's arms and share that first breath of life in the intimate bond of the family.[1]

Whether or not the father wants actually to deliver the baby as this father did, his role throughout labour can be a very positive and active one. Women who wrote about their childbirth experiences at home stressed the importance of the man attending antenatal classes and not simply being offered a special 'fathers' evening:

Peter and I said very little ... but his presence at my side was vital. I hardly looked at the midwives but depended so much on eye contact with Peter. This would not have meant much if he hadn't been to classes. He knew as well as I did what I was doing and that it was working and his confidence in me was marvellous to feel.

If a baby is to be born at home the man should understand the techniques for coping with contractions and for the varied stresses of labour, including backache, cramp, leg trembling, and overbreathing so that he can help her and use the same words and phrases as those used in the preparation the couple have received. Since few women handle every contraction with confidence it is important, too, that he has learned the breathing patterns and can do them and that he knows what relaxation means in terms of

[1] Stephen Koons: Homebirth: a family awakening. In *Safe alternatives in childbirth,* (ed. David and Lee Stewart), NAPSAC, Chapel Hill, NC (1976).

labour and how to relax at will himself. It is not enough to read a book, although valuable to do so in addition to classes.

He should also have rehearsed labour using a stressful stimulus to which the woman can adjust by conscious breathing, neuromuscular release, and focused concentration. This stressor can be a 'Chinese burn' on the forearm or pressure on the ankle but is probably most effective when it consists of a gradually increased pinch of some flesh on the inner thigh, the grip being held tightly for some 20 – 30 seconds and then decreased over a total period of 45 seconds to 2 minutes. Besides providing good practice for the pregnant woman in coping with different kinds of contractions this allows him to observe her reactions to stressful stimuli and know how to help her respond with relaxation and controlled breathing rather than involuntary tightening of muscles and panicky overbreathing. He learns to know exactly when she is most likely to contract muscles and how she can most readily be helped to let go completely. This understanding of what she looks like, her facial expression, her breathing and the sets of muscles which tend to tighten up is of great help to her in labour because he shares with her an increasing awareness of *residual* tensions. These are often cumulative in labour, being carried over from one difficult contraction to the next. They may be so slight that no one else may notice them and even the woman herself may not realize that she is tightening up. When they have practised together beforehand they will have evolved effective ways for him helping her to release tension immediately with a touch, a word, or a kiss. It is easy to get so systematized about instructions to couples about what they can or should do that the spontaneous activity taking place between a man and woman who love each other is forgotten or relegated to the background as unimportant. The outpouring of oxytocin which accompanies sexual feeling and the flood of loving emotions may do more than any techniques to help the smooth progress of dilatation and co-ordinated uterine function.

The man who is present in labour without understanding what is occurring in the woman's body and what the psychological experience may be for his wife puts himself at a disadvantage. He needs to know the nature of stressful stimuli at different phases of labour, to understand what she is feeling and share the experience in a way which is impossible for anyone who merely has a knowledge of anatomy and physiology. A sixth-form biology course is an inadequate preparation for a man who is going to participate in a labour. Even a degree course in biology does not prepare him for the reality of the experience or the emotional impact of it on him as well as on the woman who is bearing his child.

The father who has studied medicine, especially one who has done six months obstetrics, may have the necessary information about physiological processes, but in other respects he may be at an even greater disadvantage than the man who knows very little about how a woman's body works. Learning about 'the' uterus and 'the' foetus is rather different from appreciating the activity of his wife's uterus or sharing in the coming to birth of his baby. I do not think that even the most loving doctor husband is adequately prepared to help his wife or to meet the challenge of the emotional impact of birth if he does not attend classes or discussion groups during pregnancy too.

In one couple's class I was once acting the part of a woman in the late first stage encountering difficulties and losing control. I had asked the men in the room, all of whom had attended 4 or 5 meetings together already, to help me. We had previously rehearsed ways in which anyone with a woman in labour could help her handle threatening contractions. I was hyperventilating, arching my back, crying out and gripping the pillows above my head. I threshed about on the floor and had slipped flat on my back, arms and legs flailing and gasping for something to take away the pain! It happened that there was a doctor husband in the class and for some reason no one moved to come to my aid, perhaps because they were deferring to him, thinking that surely he must know the most effective action to take. After a few minutes a philosophy don came to my side, put his arms around me, sat me up and said firmly, 'Open your eyes. Look at me. Breathe with me. I'm with you', and proceeded to take charge of the situation. As the group was closing that evening the doctor came to me and said, 'I have never felt so ashamed in my life. I didn't know what to do. I realize now that I've been interested only in delivery and that I haven't a clue how to help a woman cope with the first stage.' Some weeks later he told me, 'Obstetrics is far more interesting for me now. Whenever I can I am with my patients at the end of the first stage. The thing has become really exciting!'

The man who is present at birth is not there just as hand-holder or a 'voyeur' of delivery. For his own as well as his wife's sake he needs to have a coherent role. He is there to give of his strength and love in a psychological partnership. For this he needs good preparation, adapted to the specific environment in which that birth is to take place.

II: Helping through labour: the unfolding pattern

We have already had some descriptions from women of how their partners helped them during labour. In the following pages we shall look at the main milestones of labour at home and see what a man might do when those points are reached.

OVERTURE

What happens:

May have bloody show—like beginning of period. *If steady bleeding, ring doctor.*

Low backache *or*

Indigestion-like cramps *or*

Something like a tight band of wide elastic pulling in round the lower abdomen at regular intervals 5 minutes or more apart *or*

Menstrual-like discomfort *or*

Slow leaking of bag of waters *or*

Bag of waters pops and water streams out. *Ring doctor/midwife if this happens.*

May want to pass frequent small bowel motions.

Cervix is being drawn up and thinned out (*effaced*)

What woman should do

If not sure if it is or is not labour, try completely different activity:

If in bed, get up and walk in garden/park/countryside or do some gardening or cooking.

If active, have rest and try to doze off or go out to film (can always leave when you want to).

If you have not eaten for some time have light, easily digested snack for quick energy, e.g. soup, avocado, omelette, milky drink, bread and honey, yoghurt, grapes, banana. Make sure partner eats too. If things start gently have simple meal out together in pleasant atmosphere.

Get room ready. Lighting. Flowers? Candles? Cassette tape recorder? Camera?

Birth at home

If tired, settle down in darkened room and get some sleep before labour starts in earnest. Even half an hour will refresh you.

Leave washing up.

Have bath.

If waters go, put on 2 sanitary pads and stay in own home and/or garden.

How father can help

Stay calm, confident, loving.

Check in your mind on practical arrangements, e.g. midwife and doctor's phone numbers, supplies for labour, food in house, petrol in car in case it should be needed. Make up bed together with rubber sheet, newspapers over, sheet on top of that, fresh covers on as many pillows as can be collected. See that heater is in room. Tidy and clean kitchen, dry any laundry and do basic chores round house if there might be problems about them not being done later.

Lie down and rest with wife or keep house quiet so that she has a chance of rest if this is what she wants.

Go out with her if she wants change of scene and physical activity.

If waters are leaking get her thick, clean towel.

If she wants to sit on lavatory see that room is warm.

EARLY FIRST STAGE

What happens:

Regular contractions every 5 – 10 minutes getting stronger and closer together until they are coming every 3 – 4 minutes. May follow pattern of one strong, one weak.

Possible backache/thighache.

Cervix beginning to dilate to 5 centimetres (half dilatation)

What woman should do

Carry on with gentle household work. Play with/tell stories to older child or take for walk. Upright position speeds dilatation.

Play chess/scrabble, do crosswords, read funny or gripping book, or have passages read to you.

Practise transcendental meditation, simple yoga positions and breathing.

Listen to music, play music, sing, dance, stopping to breathe way through contraction.

Do any creative activity which feels right for you.

If labour is slow invite close friends in and celebrate start.

Soak in bath.

Inform midwife when contractions lasting at least 45 seconds and coming regularly or whenever you feel right time. It helps midwife if she knows you may need her before she goes out in the morning.

During each contraction breathe slowly in through nose at beginning and out through mouth at end, and if necessary breathe more quickly and lightly over crest of contraction, through parted lips if it feels more comfortable.

120

II: Helping through labour

How father can help

Time contractions every 15 – 30 minutes, depending on frequency and write down length and interval between start of each.

Share whatever occupation she chooses.

Stop talking when contraction starts and give her your attention. Ask what she wants. Be ready to give her more air, less air, more warmth, less warmth, fresh sanitary pad, go with her to lavatory.

If older child around keep him/her happy and make any necessary arrangements for care.

Run her bath and stay near while she has it.

If she has backache offer firm pressure or, sprinkling a little talcum powder on first, rub back during contractions with *heel* of palm, fingers resting lightly on skin, or knuckles. Or get hot water bottle with cover to apply to painful area.

LATE FIRST STAGE

What happens:

Regular contractions every 2-3 minutes lasting 60 seconds or more.

Waters may go if they have not gone already.

Everything feels accelerated and more intense.

Woman becomes more serious, needs to draw on strength gained *between* contraction so wants to concentrate on her labour.

Gets irritated/impatient/apprehensive.

May feel nauseated and vomit.

Pressure against rectum and anus building up.

Cervix dilates to 8 centimetres or more.

What woman should do

Doze between contractions and relax completely.

Focus concentration on husband's face or curving shape in room or through window during contractions.

Give breath *out* as contraction is noted to greet it; then move up to breathe as lightly and rapidly as you need; mark end of contraction with resting breath, complete breath *out*.

Try the smiling butterfly breathing over peak of contraction. If breathing is quick it *must* be shallow or you will overbreathe, flush out carbon dioxide and feel giddy. It should be almost soundless.

If breathing becomes arrhythmic and you feel strained blow out crisply through lips in kissing shape, allow time for automatic breath in and carry straight on with butterfly breathing.

Find comfortable position; back, including small of back, neck, head and legs resting on firm cushions.

Midwife may offer pethidine/gas and oxygen. If using gas and oxygen apply mask firmly to face, take 2 long, slow breaths in and out through open mouth (count of about 5 seconds to each breath in and each one out) as contraction starts; then *drop* mask and go straight into butterfly breathing.

121

Birth at home

How father can help

Stay close.

Continue as earlier.

Let her know she is doing well; tell her you love her.

If she wants caresses, stroking, massage, or simply to be firmly held, do so; if she prefers to be left to concentrate on these powerful contractions to work with them, understand her need to do this.

Many women appreciate eye contact with partner during difficult contractions. If she screws up eyes, tightens neck or seems to withdraw into pain get her to open eyes and look at you and *breathe with her.*

Over mountain peaks make sure that breathing is mouth-centred and quiet as a whisper, shoulders relaxed.

Remind her that each contraction is doing good work and brings birth nearer.

Give low back pressure or massage as often as she likes it or sit on bed so that your own pelvis is pressing against small of her back.

Have bowl ready if she feels sick.

If she begins to look anxious avoid mirroring this on your face.

Smile; be positive, give quiet, loving encouragement.

Call midwife if you have not done so already.

TRANSITION

What happens:

Contractions every 1½-2 minutes may be almost continuous if each lasts 90 seconds or so; some may have double peaks.

Concentrated 'glowing', 'hot' pain at bottom of uterus as final tissues of cervix are pulled up over baby's head and baby is pressed down through it.

Signs of onset of expulsive urge: hiccups, catch in throat, involuntarily held breath, grunting, groaning on exhaled breath at end of contraction.

Legs may shake.

Feels hot/cold; lost and tossed and broken as if in tiny boat in stormy sea; may not want to be touched; increased irritability and outspokeness.

Drowsy between contractions.

May forget she is having baby.

Sensation as if there is grapefruit behind anus.

Cervix dilates to 10 centimetres, full dilatation.

What woman should do

Welcome each contraction with breath out; if difficult to keep breathing regular during contraction use blow out as if pushing balloon away from you with breath in patterned rhythm with 3 – 6 butterfly breaths followed by 1 or 2 blows; give long, full resting breath at end of each contraction so ready to start breathing with next immediately if necessary.

Use any rest-times for complete rehabilitation by dropping against pillows and releasing any tension.

II: Helping through labour

Relax buttocks, pelvic floor spread down, heavy like loaded hammock.

How father can help

Remind her of all signs of progress and that baby will be in her arms before
long.

Continue giving emotional support as for late first stage. She may
appreciate sponge down with cool/hot water.

May like hot water bottle between legs, at feet, in small of back.

Change of position can be helpful; she may feel rooted to bed so needs to
be moved (between contractions).

May appreciate firm holding or massage. If she is shaking firm massage of
both inner thighs can be useful; use whole palm of each hand, fingers
pointing down and massage down from top of inside legs to knees and
light stroke back up over top of legs, keeping continuous, rhythmic
movement; if on her side she may like firm buttock massage as if
kneading bread dough, but keeping hands still and using fingers.

Be generous with praise, give information; you are her anchor in a stormy
sea.

Offer sips of cold water and ice to suck between contractions; vaseline or
lipsalve for lips.

Maintain quietness in room during each contraction and peaceful
atmosphere.

THE 'REST AND BE THANKFUL' INTERVAL

What happens:

Contractions may get weak or fade away for anything from 5 to 20 minutes
following full dilatation of cervix.

What woman should do

Rest; close your eyes and enjoy the peace.

How father can help

Brush her hair back from eyes, wash face. Offer cologne or toilet water.

Put out baby clothes, warm nappies in front of fire; check room is warm
for baby.

Soft, relaxing music?

Relax and wait patiently for resumption of uterine activity.

SECOND STAGE

What happens

Powerful urges to bear down and press baby through birth canal occur in
waves 1 – 4 times during each contraction; may feel as if *being pushed*
rather than pushing.

Anal pressure may feel preposterous; changes to vaginal distension as
second stage progresses with tingling, stretching, hot sensation.

May have small bowel movement and/or a little more blood may appear
when pushing.

Birth at home

What woman should do

Experiment with posture until it feels right. Try sitting up, kneeling, squatting, on all fours.

Right time to push is when you *want* to; do what comes naturally, trust your feelings.

During contractions continue light, quick breathing through relaxed mouth except when breath spontaneously held as desire to push is at height; then hold breath, keeps lips parted; breathe again in little, short breaths as soon as you can.

Drop head forward during contraction; keep mouth loose and soft; relax shoulders, legs, and feet.

Enjoy fullness and heaviness against pelvic floor and press muscles down and forward during pushing like a lift which is going down to basement.

Shift position so that whoever is catching baby can reach you easily; usually means sliding buttocks forward so that you are sitting on base of spine or lying on side, back rounded, for left lateral delivery.

Put hands down to feel top of baby's head in vagina and whole head when it has slipped out.

As head stretches vulva stop pushing and start breathing so that baby is breathed out rather than suddenly ejected. Think with each breath 'out, out, out' or 'open, open, open'.

Reach out arms for baby and do whatever you feel like doing.

Hold naked baby against your skin.

How father can help

Prop her up well or help her adjust position so that upper part of body is well raised; any position in which she is most comfortable is right one; kneeling or sitting behind her so that back and shoulders are supported may be good.

If midwife not present be ready with soft cotton wool balls soaked in boiled water to which antiseptic added and gently wipe down and away from vagina if she needs her bottom wiped; have pedal bin near bed for disposal. Sponge her with cold water; offer ice chips between contractions.

Encourage her by saying 'open up' and 'good', not 'push'.

Tell her if you can see head and adjust mirror so that she can see.

May like to receive baby in your hands and/or to cut cord; can suggest this to midwife.

At delivery greet baby. Let feelings flow!

AFTERWARDS

What happens

Placenta and membranes will be delivered within 45 minutes or so. Contractions renewed for this.

Bleeding should only be about ½ pint.

May feel ravenous.

II: Helping through labour

What woman should do

Cuddle baby.

Watch for when baby opens eyes—Marvellous moment!

Suckle baby.

Bear down to expel placenta. Ask midwife to show it if interested.

Massage uterus.

How father can help

If alone do not cut cord. Leave till placenta is delivered.

Cover mother and baby with light warm covering.

Help baby onto breast when he/she begins to root for nipple.

Make tea for mother and midwife. Get food.

Care for other child.

Celebrate!

9

The birthday

I am tired of being told I am brave to have my babies at home. It is simply that I like my husband, my friend the midwife, my roses, my curtains and my cracked ceiling about me to give me confidence and no distraction when I have a hard day's work to do.

THIS chapter aims to discover what labour and delivery at home may be like. It is based on accounts by 65 women who lived in different parts of Britain and some others in the USA and Australia, all of whom had decided to have their babies at home. Since every labour is unique and the subjective experience of childbirth varies widely it is important that the woman who is expecting a baby does not approach the birth with a picture in her mind of how she feels labour *ought* to be but is able to accept it as it is.

Labour may begin 40 weeks following the first day of the last menstrual period, but it equally well may not. Any time within two weeks before or after this estimated date of delivery is common and if labour starts in this 4-week period the baby is born 'at term'. One of the women who wrote a lengthy account of her home birth went apparently 5 weeks overdue and said:

Kathryn was originally due on September 12th but she was born on October 20th. I was allowed to go for so long overdue as it was later decided that I had not conceived until 4 weeks after my last period. I had only one period after coming off the Pill and the cycle had not returned to normal.

Those last 5 weeks were very worrying as I felt threatened at the thought of having to be admitted to hospital for induction and my GP and midwife knew this. My voice quivered and hands shook whenever they mentioned it!

If a woman becomes pregnant shortly after coming off the pill as this woman did, her pregnancy can often not be dated with certainty. It helps if she can note carefully her first awareness of foetal movement, which usually happens at about 16 weeks.

Birth at home

First labours often last 15 or 16 hours, second and subsequent labours are often about half that length. But at least half of a slowly unfolding labour is likely to be of the kind where the woman can carry on almost as normal, and in fact she labours better if she is up and about.

Labour can start in different ways, with regular, rhythmic tightenings, the contractions, which get longer, closer together and more powerful over several hours; with a bloody 'show' as the mucus plug comes away from the cervix, which forms the opening of the uterus; by rupture of the membranes or bag of waters; occasionally just by a dull backache or a feeling as if one were about to begin a menstrual period; sometimes a thighache or an apparent gastrointestinal disturbance. The show can occur several weeks ahead of labour, however, so although it is a sign that the uterus is getting ready for the work of labour, it is not an indication that it has started.

Regular contractions which get progressively stronger and come more and more frequently are a much more reliable indication that labour has begun. The uterus is an enormous muscle and each contraction pulls together, shortens and squeezes the muscle fibres. When this happens anyone with a hand resting over the uterus, the father or the mother herself, can feel it is hard. If the father looks at the abdominal profile during a contraction he can see that the upper part is tilted forward and with a strong contraction it looks as if the whole abdominal wall is swelling with the tremendous force liberated behind it.

The outer layer of muscle which runs from top to bottom of the uterus is pulling up and gradually drawing open the cervix at the lower end, and at the same time the baby is being steadily pressed down towards this opening. The only sure sign that one really is in labour is progressive dilatation of the cervix. This softening, stretching, thinning out and opening of the cervix so that the baby's head can pass through it is what is achieved by the work of the uterus throughout the first stage of labour. The cervix needs to dilate to 10 centimetres before it is fully open and the baby can be pressed down to delivery. Many women start off labour already 2 centimetres or more dilated because contractions in the last weeks of pregnancy have had a softening and then a dilating effect on the cervix.

Two of the mothers who wrote started off labour with the waters breaking. One found herself leaking 2 weeks before labour started. When waters go early like this obstetricians are concerned about possible pelvic infection unless the baby is delivered within 24 hours, but this woman refused to go into hospital: 'I was stuck at home going mad. Everyone did their best to get me into hospital for antibiotics, induction, etc. It was awful!' But after 2 weeks her baby engaged in the pelvis 'and away we went' into an easy, straightforward labour.

All the other women began labour by realizing that they were having contractions, often had a show as well and described how they carried on with household activities, read, watched television, went for a walk, baked a cake, washed their hair, did some gardening, looked after their other children, or entertained friends. Some lay in a warm bath for a long time and found it easy to relax there. Others had several baths at intervals. One woman planted runner beans, stopping only to relax and 'breathe deliberately' with each contraction. 'When labour starts', said one woman, 'there is no upheaval, having to rush out into the cold night, find somewhere to park the children, etc. You can carry on as normal and go to bed when you feel like it.' Another woman described how after the waters had begun to leak and she had had contractions at 10-minute intervals for 4 hours which then died away, she went out to supper with her husband, and then to bed for a 'good few hours sleep' before labour began in earnest.

Many women referred to the advantages of being in one's own home and one's own bed, in familiar, comfortable surroundings. 'Labour seemed much shorter', one woman commented, 'because I didn't go upstairs until I got to the stage of feeling if I didn't go up soon I wouldn't manage the stairs'. A woman who said, 'There is no need for the expectant mother to change her usual daily routine or go to bed until she feels like it, so that birth seems a much shorter process', added that: 'It may actually be shorter, if the relaxation possible in the comfort and security of one's own home allows physical processes to proceed with less interference.'

Not one of the 65 went to lie on the bed until labour was well established and contractions coming so thick and fast that she felt she had to stop everything else. Even then women often preferred to be other than in bed and referred to an especially comfortable chair or sofa which was suitable for much of the first stage of labour: 'The midwife came, found me crouching over a beanbag reading *The life and death of Marilyn Monroe*. . . . When my legs twitched too much to walk about in between [contractions], she got me into bed.'

The decision to call the midwife was usually made only after contractions were coming close together, although many women warned the midwife that they thought something was happening well in advance and she often visited to assess the situation and see that the mother was comfortable, leaving phone numbers where she could be found before she went on her rounds.

The midwife arrived and said I was 'about 2 fingers[1] plus dilated'. She saw that Derrick and I were obviously coping very well and asked if we minded her going off on a few urgent calls. Of course we didn't. I pottered around the house all morning, feeling so excited!

Women were often especially grateful for the skilled and understanding care they received from their midwives:

As in art, simplicity is only achieved by a great deal of thorough preparation and work. The professionalism and attention to detail of my midwife and the whole domiciliary service (including my very pro-home-confinement GP) cannot be praised too highly and I feel in many respects the service and attention of the domiciliary team is of a higher standard, on a purely medical level, than it is in some hospitals.

Meeting a new midwife when in labour because the one they were used to was away on holiday was not only stressful for those women who had this experience, but actually sometimes threatened emotional control. It happened to few women, fortunately, largely because community midwives were eager to attend a home birth even when they were off duty and willingly gave up free time. It seemed that the midwives had an emotional investment in their patients no less than they relied on their midwives to be with them.

But a new step on the landing, a strange face, however friendly, a different voice, filled some women with a momentary sense of panic:

The midwife arrived with a pupil midwife. We had met her for the first time that morning and had to explain about classes and discuss our plans in about 10 minutes whereas I had been working on my own midwife for months. . . I told her that I did not like pethidine. . .

Discussing analgesics with someone they had not met before was often difficult.

[1] 4 centimetres: double the number of fingers to assess dilatation

The birthday

Women often chose not to have their perineal hair shaved and many did not have an enema, two of the routine procedures which they frequently disliked about previous hospital births.

I was very grateful that there was no question of tampering with me, no enemas, no shaving, no cutting, no drugs; we were both so thankful not to have to waste any energy in arguing the toss over any of these things.

One woman who was having her first baby with a GP and midwife who both enjoyed home deliveries wrote:

At 10 a.m. I had a show and was so relieved something positive had happened at last. I had had imaginary signs for weeks! Nick was just as excited by the news as he was tired of waiting too. Contractions then came every 10 minutes although I wondered if they were *labour* pains as they seemed much milder than I had expected. About 1 p.m. I began to feel I needed to breathe through them and did not want to talk during them. At 4.30 they were coming every 5 minutes and lasting 30 seconds but still the pain was mild. At 6 I rang the midwife. She said she'd see me in an hour but to ring if I needed her. I felt very relaxed and did some quick revision of the NCT leaflet. The midwife arrived at 7 p.m. I had an enema, which achieved nothing, and a bath. She examined me and I was 2 fingers dilated but not enough for her to break the membranes. She left and I went downstairs to watch the TV. She told me to ring her at 10 p.m. This I did by which time the contractions were lasting 45 seconds and coming at 5 minute intervals. They were not consistently strong, but I seemed to get a strong one and less strong one alternately.

This mother's account illustrates the normal progress of a labour which started fairly slowly. If she had gone into hospital in the morning when contractions were coming every 10 minutes, as women are often instructed to do, she would probably have been put to bed and since many obstetricians today consider a prolonged and hence abnormal labour is one that lasts more than 12 hours, or sometimes more than 10 or even 8 hours, she might well have had her labour accelerated with an oxytocin drip and have had no choice about it. As it was she had a spontaneous delivery, with no analgesia, and no episiotomy.

When contractons are first noticed there may be as much as 10 minutes between them, but they gradually get closer together till they are coming every 2 minutes, or sometimes even closer. The baby will not be born until they are coming that frequently. The contractions also frequently start with each lasting about 45 seconds or less, and they become longer so that when the end of the first stage is reached, they may last 1½ or even 2 minutes, and there is scarcely any pause between them.

Sometimes they come regularly and frequently but do not last long. It is usually only when each contraction lasts about a minute that the cervix is completely opened so that the baby's head is pressing down in the birth canal. The woman in the above account had very short contractions, even though they were coming every 5 minutes, until her labour had been going for 12 hours or more.

The midwife usually told the mother how much the cervix was dilated after each vaginal examination. From Fig 4 on pp. 134 – 5 the woman in labour can see exactly how far she is dilated.

Sometimes the first stage drags on a long time and the mother becomes progressively more tired. Fatigue makes it more difficult for her to cope with the contractions and she tends to feel pain more readily. Occasionally, too, contractions get feeble or stop altogether for a time. In hospital the labour is then accelerated or augmented (both terms mean the same thing) with an oxytocin intravenous drip. This often leads to strong pain killers having to be given to enable the mother to tolerate the forceful, rapidly recurring contractions, for as one obstetrician explains it: 'Women with augmented labour do need stronger doses of drugs for relief of pain. Possibly the ideal method for them is an epidural anaesthetic started soon after the commencement of the labour. If the epidural is properly administered and is . . . effective the labour will not only be more rapid but also painless. There will then, however, be a greater need for forceps delivery.'[1]

Clearly this sequence of events cannot take place at home. It is dangerous to administer oxytocin at home because the effect on the uterus cannot be known in advance, and the sophisticated equipment necessary for monitoring the foetal heart and the contractions throughout is not available. But the woman labouring at home can do several things to get the uterus working more effectively: she can get up and walk about, go in the garden for example, or move around while listening to music. Or if she prefers to rest she can change position on a pile of cushions or a bean bag on the floor and kneel, squat or get onto all fours. Whatever position she finds most comfortable is likely to be the best one for her and tends to tilt the baby into the right position.

Equally, if not even more important than any postural variations

[1] Elliot Philipp: *Childbirth*, Fontana, London (1978).

or comfort techniques are the woman's spontaneous feelings about the experience of birth and these in turn depend a good deal on the attitudes of everyone around her and whether or not they are anxious when contractions seem to be weak or ineffective. When I was working in the hills in Jamaica I learned that the folk midwives encountering secondary uterine inertia in an exhausted mother would massage her with oil from the castor oil plant and then wrap her in hot towels and let her rest until contractions picked up in strength again. This treatment was often remarkably effective.

Oxytocin is released into the blood stream during sexual excitement and it is endogenous oxytocin which usually stimulates the already sensitive uterus into activity. This may explain why loving caresses between a couple during labour may have a positive effect on the progress of dilatation and why when secondary inertia occurs love-making can often trigger off uterine activity again. Nipple stimulation is particularly effective, but perhaps the way in which it is done and by whom it is done is even more important than the fact that it is done. Nipple stimulation is sometimes performed mechanically in certain hospitals in studies to find out whether or not it produces release of oxytocin. In one study[1] it was discovered that an electric breast pump used for 15 minutes on each breast alternately could actually induce labour in 71 per cent of women, and after rupture of the membranes could do so in 79 per cent of cases. Women whose babies were postmature started labour in 63 per cent of cases. When uterine inertia occurred after labour was established 95 per cent of women started contractions again. Nipple stimulation was slightly more effective in women having second or subsequent babies than in those having a first baby. Contractions started within 3 hours in 55 per cent of multigravidae and 39 per cent of primigravidae.

At home this can be done by the woman's partner as part of their normal relationship and his active, loving sharing in the labour which is giving birth to their child, and this can include kissing mouth to mouth, nipple sucking, and clitoral stimulation if the couple enjoy this. Only those acts should be performed which the woman enjoys and all mechanical procedures should be absolutely ruled out. It might be the right moment for the midwife to go down to the kitchen and get herself a cup of tea!

[1] A. Jhivad and T. Vaog: Induction of labor by breast stimulation. *Contemporary Obstetrics and Gynecology:* 109 – 13 (1974).

Birth at home

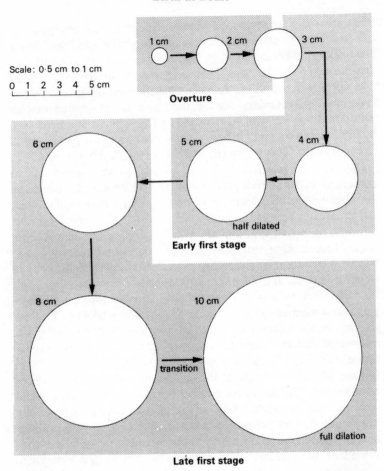

FIG. 4. Dilatation of the cervix during labour.

Throughout labour the midwife monitors the foetal heart rate. Babies who are going to need help with breathing have always suffered distress in labour: problems after birth do not appear out of the blue.

Women who had their babies at home often said they appreciated the absence of medical mystique and that they were kept fully informed of progress, delay, good signs, and difficulties. Two women had unfortunate experiences, however, because midwives in their area were not accustomed to doing home

134

The birthday

deliveries and were frightened by the responsibility. In each case staff from the hospital arrived in the home to conduct the labour. One woman wrote:

All midwives are based at our hospital. So at 2 a.m. when I felt I was having strong contractions I felt I ought to phone the hospital to let someone know. My husband had to go and fetch the midwives from the hospital (I suppose they were without cars). On his arrival there the Night Sister greeted him with 'Couldn't you persuade her to come in? It would be much safer.' . . . A Sister came with a pupil midwife who was thrilled to bits and subsequently wrote me up for her finals. . . . It was good to be at home, but if there can be such a thing it was a hospitalized home confinement. They turned our bedroom into a hospital. Everything was timed, recorded, methodical, sterile. They were worried about what would happen if I were still in labour when they should go off duty. They reported (on the telephone) back to the hospital that they wouldn't give me much longer, and I knew that meant forceps and I knew that forceps meant hospital. I must have been frightened into pushing harder and Danielle was born at 7 a.m.

It is a sad reflection on the present state of midwifery training and on the lack of knowledge about the normal progress of undrugged, unaugmented labour or of experience in home deliveries that the midwife in this account became anxious and allowed this anxiety to be communicated to the mother.

Most of the midwives, however, seemed delighted to have the opportunity to do a home birth and treated it as a special privilege. Some of the midwives who enjoyed home births remarked that it is an experience which is often denied pupil midwives so that sometimes they qualify without ever having seen a completely natural birth.

Women often expressed deep gratitude to their midwives. One mother, commenting on her 'peaceful, contented baby', said that she thought she was like this because she was 'born in a very peaceful, happy atmosphere:

I was in control, I was in my own bed (where I had been born, in fact!) in my own home, and I didn't feel 'taken over' by a vast body of people in white masks. Traditionally birth was never a mysterious activity to be carried out in hospitals under the supervision of men. It was an essential part of the role of women which took place in the baby's home amid the comfort of friends and relations.

Birth at home

During labour more show appears at intervals, looking rather like bleeding in the early stage of a menstrual period. The mother should not be bleeding continually and heavily. If this should happen, get her to a hospital.

As contractions become more intense, longer, and closer together the labouring woman may feel caught up in a timeless dream which seems as if it will never end. It is also a task which demands all her energy to meet each contraction wave and 'swim' over it with her breathing.

If the waters have not gone already they may start to leak or may pop now. The fluid should be clear. Any staining from the meconium in the baby's bowels can indicate foetal distress, which is a sign that delivery should follow soon. If this happens when the second stage is still apparently a good way off the woman should be moved to hospital, or the obstetrician called since a forceps delivery may be necessary.

Once contractions are coming every 2 or 3 minutes the labouring woman may have little idea of when labour began, of how long it has lasted, or whether or not there is any progress. She may even forget that she is going to have a baby, so enormous is the undertaking, so compelling and absorbing that she can only give her whole self to each moment. At the end of the first stage, between 7 and 10 centimetres dilatation, there may be only a brief pause before the next contraction comes like a great wave following on the last. The women feels as if she is swimming in a stormy sea and it can be frightening, awesome, exciting, painful, and joyous. She needs all her concentration, her sense of purpose and courage, and the loving support and encouragement of those with her.

Several women emphasized that their labours were painful at the end of the first stage, but stressed that they preferred to experience this in the comfort of their own beds in their own homes with a friendly midwife helping and their husbands present than in the alien environment of a hospital.

It is at this phase of labour that the woman may start to shake, her legs to twitch and she may hiccup, belch or suddenly vomit. Though disconcerting, they are all signs of progress. The first stage is reaching its climax and soon the second stage will start, when the baby can be pushed out.

Readers who would like to find out more about the unfolding patterns of labour, how to assess progress, how the mother can prepare herself in advance, and techniques for coping with contractions should read *The experience of childbirth*.[1]

Here is how one woman who had been to my own childbirth classes described the end of the first stage:

Despite all the preparations and rehearsals several things surprised us. 1. That no two contractions were alike. . . . 2. The enormous amount of concentration necessary. . . . 3. Most amazing, the breathing and relaxation really worked. We never gave analgesia a thought! Breathing in labour was so easy compared to rehearsals, just a case of listening to the contraction and doing what seemed right. During the late 1st stage I improvised with butterfly breathing and crisp blowing out. I did experience an 'unreal' stage but recognised it for what it was as did Dick who sponged me over with ice cold water. It helped to remember to keep my eyes open during contractions . . . and to keep my 'singer's face' on, a step away from smiling . . . I depended so much on my eye contact with Dick.

Another did not find the breathing exercises she had learned in antenatal classes helped because 'they made me feel I was withdrawing from the centre of activity, so that I was in one place whilst the pain was running amok in another and getting on top of me'. So she invented a different breathing pattern which felt right for her: 'I found it easier . . . to stay with the pain as it washed around and in doing this I found that the pain was surprisingly localized.'

The woman having her baby at home is unlikely to be lying flat as she often is in hospital and may be able to choose which position she prefers. There is a strong case to be made for an upright posture in which the natural forces of gravity can help the descent of the baby and one in which intra-abdominal pressure allows her to ease out the child steadily and without wasted effort. The most effective position is one in which she is sitting up, the least effective positions those in which she is lying down on her back or side. In one study of intra-abdominal pressure produced in different positions it was discovered that a woman could produce 30.5 per cent more pressure onto a balloon in her vagina connected to a mercury manometer when sitting up than when lying down on her side.[1] This is because the weight of her own internal organs helps to build up pressure when the upper part of her body is well raised and because

---

[1] Sheila Kitzinger: Penguin, Harmondsworth (6th edn: 1978).

[2] See Mangert and Murphy as referred to in Richard J. Atwood: Parturitional posture and related birth behavior . . . *Acta Obstetrica et Gynecologica Scandinavica*, Supplement 57 (1976).

there can be much more efficient muscular action (as anyone can test if they try to empty their bowels lying flat). Some women like to kneel or squat or to get on all fours. The right position for any woman is the one which is comfortable for her at the time.

The urge to push may come with startling force and suddenness or may slowly build up in intensity. Many women described the sensation as irresistible and compelling in its sheer physical power. A woman who had a very rapid second stage of only several contractions wrote:

There was a sudden overwhelming pushing contraction. I got in a good position and tried to concentrate on all we had learned for 2nd stage. Everything happened too quickly with the midwives still scrubbing up and the head coming down fast. I had three pushing contractions with fairly long spaces in between. My thighs got cramp in the final contraction. . . . Then the head was out. With another contraction Rose was delivered, gargling mucus, slippy, wet and lovely on my tummy.

A woman who had a 35-minute second stage described it this way:

I experienced what seemed like a transition type contraction, having a pushing sensation as well as a 1st stage contraction. I told the midwife and asked her if it could be Transition as it seemed to have come too soon. There was then a lot of activity in the room and the GP arrived. He is a very calm person and his presence had a reassuring effect on me. I was using the Huff Huff Puff Puff breathing. I was told I could push which again surprised me as I had expected to have to wait much longer for the privilege. I didn't find 2nd stage contractions compelling and I found it really hard work but I had a great feeling of determination. . . . I didn't think I was making any progress until Paul shouted that he could see the baby's head. The Doctor told me that things were being held up as the cord was round her neck and that it was being removed. A few more hard pushes and she was born . . . I just felt totally relaxed and happy and united with Paul. I just lay there enjoying a marvellous sense of achievement.

Another woman almost had a forceps delivery:

The second stage started at 10 p.m. and I felt completely in control and very happy. I suspected nothing wrong when the Midwife asked my husband to phone the doctor about three quarters of an hour later. The Duty Doctor, unfortunately not my GP, arrived about ten minutes later, and the Midwife quietly suggested that I was going to need a forceps delivery. However I was determined to do it all myself this time, which I did while the forceps were being sterilized, only five minutes after the doctor's arrival. I almost heard a fanfare of trumpets as the head crowned. It was the most marvellous moment when the little wet body slipped between my thighs.

As the baby's head stretches the perineal tissues they fan out in response to its pressure. The woman feels first a sensation of bulging against her anus so that she may think she wants to empty her bowels, and then a stretching, tingling feeling around her vagina. With the first sensation it is important that she goes on pushing whenever she has the urge to do so, pressing the baby down towards the anus and not trying to 'hold it in'. When the second sensation comes she should relax completely, feeling herself soft and loose below, parting her lips and feeling the vagina also open and soft, and breathe in and out through her open mouth as she lets the baby be born with her *breathing* rather than her pushing. The head can then ooze out without strain and the likelihood of a tear or of requiring an episiotomy is much reduced.

It is important that the mother and her midwife work together so that the baby's head glides out slowly and steadily rather than exploding from the vagina. Ina May of the Farm in Tennessee expresses this cooperation as 'mind-contact' and says:

> Sometimes, while helping a mother through crowning, I feel like I'm outside a semi-trailer truck, directing the driver: 'All right, bring it on a little now—hold it for a few seconds now, Okay, bring it on some more.' You can get a very telephathic thing going with the mother . . . and while she holds back that tremendous force, the whole quality of her skin will change—she will relax and become more pliant and stretchy.[1]

Women having their babies at home often put their hands down to touch the head before the baby is born. Some describe how they feel the top of the head even before the rest of it has slipped out. Those who did so found that doing this made the extraordinary sensations produced by the pressure of the head on the perineum much easier to cope with and they often said that this experience was particularly exciting because for the first time they were in contact with the emerging baby. It is easy to believe that you are not having a baby at all when you push and nothing seems to happen! Easy to forget the existence of the baby, too, when your whole body and mind is caught up in the incredible power and energy of pushing contractions. Those mothers who reached down

[1] Ina May Gaskin: *Spiritual midwifery.* Book Publishing Co., The Farm, Summertown, Tennessee (1978).

and felt the baby even before the head crowned spoke of their wonder and joy at what was for them a precious moment of realization that here was the baby who was soon to be in their arms.

Some community midwives as a matter of practice suggest to mothers that they do this and may tell the mother to reach down and hold her baby and help lift it from her own body. There is no reason why this should not be done in hospital and some midwives do so. But in practice, so many more women in hospital are 'zonked out' with drugs or are watching in a mirror an occurrence happening at the lower end of a body which has no feeling in it because of epidural anaesthesia, that mothers seem to be less ready to do this, and in the hospital obstetric delivery with its carefully co-ordinated team work between professionals, obstetricians and midwives tend to be the active deliverers while the mothers are relatively passive, acted on rather than active. If this is to happen more frequently we need to change the management of delivery and see the relationship between the mother and her baby starting even before the child is delivered and handed to her.

Some of the women who wrote wanted the baby to be delivered gently according to the teaching of Frédérick Leboyer, and they usually found midwives were interested and flexible in their approach to adapt to mothers' wishes. Some explained that they always did things that way and felt that it was important for the baby to be spared any unnecessary shock, to be handed straight to the mother and to lie in her arms. The discussions reported between mothers and midwives reminded me of the birth of my own twins, when the midwife was regretful that she did not have time to prepare a warm bath into which to deliver the babies. I asked her why she did this, and she explained that since a baby had been lying in water inside the uterus she always put a bowl of water between the mother's legs and placed the newborn baby in it straight away. She thought that this eased the shock of birth and that babies seemed happier once they were in the familiar water again.

One woman wrote:

Our feelings about childbirth are very much in accordance with Dr. Leboyer's philosophy, and I feel that his teaching is very enlightened and valuable. The midwives dutifully acquainted themselves with Dr. Leboyer's book, which we bought them specially for the purpose, and they were generally open to all the Leboyer-type requests which we made of them.

The birthday

One mother commented on the way in which 'so much of what people are now saying ought to be done at birth for babies was done quite spontaneously':

I put him to the breast straight away. He was bathed. There were no harsh lights and loud noises. I was relaxed and comfortable. He fed well and slept well, was laughing by 10 days, loves life generally. Who knows, he may well have been like that after a tricky forceps delivery in a cold well-lit hospital delivery room, but I can't help feeling. . . .

After the delivery the baby was always handed straight to the mother, and often remained in her arms through the third stage of labour, when the delivery of the placenta takes place, and was suckled as soon as it rooted for the nipple:

I was given Hilary almost immediately while they dealt with the placenta. When she had been bathed she was returned to me to feed. She suckled straight away. I was thrilled with her. She had no marks on her or any redness as I had expected she would and I thought she was beautiful. When everyone had left and she had been put in her crib, she wouldn't settle so I lifted her out and I lay awake nursing her for the rest of the night. Neither of us had experienced such complete happiness ever before.

When it comes to the point of actually handing over their babies to be bathed according to the Leboyer ritual some mothers found it very difficult to part with them, even though the bathing was to be done in the same room. They felt that the right place for their babies to be was against their own bodies and even the bath represented precious minutes lost from this first personal contact with the newborn.

It is clear that mothers who have their babies at home feel that they want their babies with them and that they know what to do for them better than anybody else. This may be because the women are those most likely to choose and persevere to have home birth. It may also be that birth at home sets off powerful emotional releasers for intense interaction with the baby.

A number of mothers, and fathers too, who had intended that the baby should be born in quietness according to the teachings of Leboyer, forgot all about this in their excitement and shouted with joy. They described how they laughed and wept, hugged each other, repeated phrases over and over again, and the mother sometimes said that she 'grabbed' her child or, for example, held on to him 'fiercely'. It was all part of an intensely passionate

141

experience in which there was no possibility of hushed whispers. Both parents were caught up in something for which premeditated actions and speech seemed irrelevant.

I believe it is important to note this, for birth is essentially a psychosexual experience and can be for both parents. Leboyer focuses attention on the need for babies to be greeted and welcomed into the world with consideration and gentleness, handled as people rather than hunks of flesh.

This message is vital for us today, when techniques and technology have often taken over from personal interaction and human caring. Yet the Leboyer teaching can be ritualized and turned into yet another method, as if somehow being quiet at delivery, turning down the lights and then putting the baby in a bath makes everything else all right.

The baby is born as a person and is to grow up in a family. His birthright is to participate in the human experience from the first moments of life. This experience involves powerful emotions and 'gut' reactions. It is clear from the way in which mothers write about home birth, and from my own personal experience of five home births, that birth is an act of love. Like all love-making it has its own imperatives, which sweep through and shape all the behaviour of those who are caught up in it so that the senses are sharpened and it feels as if every single cell in the body and all awareness serves the purpose of this one activity.

The baby's birth and welcome into life is part of this rich experience, not something that can start during special 'bonding time' allowed after the chores of delivery are completed. If the labour and delivery have themselves been conducted in a warm, loving atmosphere and the woman has felt that she can safely do what she feels like doing, she spontaneously greets her baby in the right way. She does not need to be taught how to do it. No elaborate plans need be made. The midwife and doctor who, in the words of one hospital Director of Nursing, consider that it is necessary to 'provide a bond between the mother and baby and other members of the family' might be rather confused at the sequence of events which was taking place and find it difficult to record and to assess their relative importance. For when a mother takes her newborn baby up on to her body in flesh-to-flesh contact it is an integral part of the sexual act of birthing, and everything she says and does then, the compassion and tenderness, the wonder and awe, the ecstatic utterance, the laughter and tears, the often fierce possessiveness, the way she touches and explores her baby, are all part of this essentially sexual experience.

The time immediately following delivery was also important for these mothers who gave birth at home. Most of them had had no drugs and felt very awake, with minds racing, in a heightened state of acute awareness for some hours after the delivery. This contrasts with the dulled mental state of any woman who has received the narcotic drugs which are frequently used in hospital and which are also employed in higher dosages than those given at home. In hospital, too, women who were awake and excited were often made to take sleeping pills after delivery and missed this important time during which the birth is relived and the new relationship with the baby dawns in its reality.

One woman, for example, wrote that she 'couldn't sleep with sheer happiness that night, as my tiny baby lay beside me in her cradle.' After her previous birth it had taken six months before she felt she had 'built up a good relationship' and the baby had been 'difficult'. This time she had:

no postnatal depression, established a good relationship with the baby and found it gently easy to slip back into normal household routine. One of the best things about this confinement was the gradual easing off of the postnatal support given by doctor and midwife. The Health Visitor called and said that she and the Midwife had an agreement whereby the Midwife continued to look after 'her' babies where possible. After my official signing off, the Midwife continued to call, first weekly, then fortnightly and finally about once a month until the baby was around a year old.

Many commented on the excellent postnatal care:

I found the postnatal nursing by the district midwives more comprehensive than the attention and advice available to mothers at local hospitals. . . . Several friends seem to have enjoyed the 'sixth-form dormitory' atmosphere in hospital whereas I enjoyed the individual attention and freedom of actions at home.

All the mothers breastfed and all without exception indicated that they enjoyed interacting with their babies in the first days and weeks after delivery, often in contrast to their experience after previous hospital deliveries. 'My baby has been close to me from the very start', said one woman, 'in both the physical and emotional sense and I can only attribute it to the process of childbirth which was normal, natural and enjoyable, as it ought to be.' Another, remarking on the way in which a home birth had 'fulfilled a dream', wrote that her baby was thriving and content and she felt that his obvious happiness must have something to do with the joy of the home birth and the gentleness with which he had been introduced to life.

Yet another wrote:

This delivery was so much exactly what a birth should be like, and it made such a strong impression and has given me such an 'easy', confident person of a baby that I shall always be grateful. . . . The point I would like to make is not that it was an earth-shattering experience but almost the opposite—a simple, straightforward event that happened naturally as part of the rhythm of the day (labour took place, very conveniently, between lunch and tea on a Sunday afternoon!)

All the women who planned to have more babies hoped that they would be able to have these at home too. This tallies with studies in which women's preferences have been investigated, in all of which it is clear that there is a large section of the population which would choose birth at home if given the opportunity. Goldthorp and Richman's study[1] of women who, although booked for hospital, had to have home delivery because of a strike in the National Health Service, indicated that a large majority of women preferred home, and this independently of whether the labour at home had been easy or difficult.

Almost every woman who wrote to me commented on the effect that birth at home had on the later relationship between her and the baby, and not only between them, but also between the father and his baby.

Birth is not only the dramatic climax of pregnancy. It is not simply the process of getting a baby out of a woman's body. It is an experience which can have significance and intrinsic value for the woman, the father of the child, and the whole family. The meaning that birth has for the couple who are becoming parents and their active participation in it may be important for their development as a man and woman able to father and mother and to derive pleasure from it.

Bonding of mother, father, and baby is not just a question of what happens in the minutes *after* birth, but of the whole

[1] W. O. Goldthorp and J. Richman: Maternal attitudes to unintended home confinement. *Practitioner* **212**, 845 (1974).

environment in which labour takes place. It is not a chemical which can be injected into parents after delivery to enable them to become effective care-givers. It is the result of a slow and powerful process started in pregnancy, made more intense when foetal movements are recognized and both parents begin to get to know their baby while it is still inside the uterus, and continued through labour in which the woman is free to find her own rhythms, express her sexuality, and *be herself* without constraint or inhibition, and in which the man is also free to express his own emotions and become not just an onlooker but a father.

Birth then becomes a celebration of life.

Postscript

I started this book by talking about the importance of being able to choose between alternatives and make decisions about our bodies and health care, and wanting to record what many women had told me about their experience of home births. In my own births, all at home, I have experienced deep joy and I am sure that the delight I have felt must have spilled over into what I have written, with the result that some readers may think I am trying to persuade people to have home births. This has not been my intention. For me the important thing is education to understand our own bodies and our lives better (psychological education, not a mere amassing of facts) and freedom of choice to decide between alternatives. Some will choose one way, some another; some will want hospital and others home; some women will want epidurals and hope not to feel anything and others will long to give birth feeling everything. I believe that a vital part of the free society we are trying to create is that each individual should have opportunity to develop their own inner potential and take responsibility for their own actions and decisions.

The task of the maternity services is to ensure that as many babies as possible can be born physically perfect. But there is more to having a baby than that. Babies are born to women; but they need to grow up in families. I believe that the environment for birth should be a suitable setting for a profound psychosexual experience, for the bonding not only between mother and baby but also between father and baby and for the spontaneous unfolding interaction between them which gives birth to a new *family*.

For those women who are able to give birth naturally as part of a spontaneous physiological process in which obstetric intervention is not necessary hospital will only be better than home when, and if, it can provide such an environment more effectively. The creation of an up-to-date home-birth service is an important function of the health services in a responsible society.

Bibliography

SOME books and other materials which may help you to decide what kind of birth to seek. There is a great mixture here, including psychology, journalism, books on methods of preparation for childbirth, books by mothers about their personal experiences, feminist books, those written by doctors for mothers, and obstetric textbooks. It is not suggested that you need to read all of them. They are additional to references in the text.

If you are pregnant you may decide that reading about obstetric pathology is not a good idea. If you do want to read an obstetric book, remember that it is focused on disease and physiological malfunction rather than health and normality. I think it is best to borrow it from a library, and not to have it hanging round the house in late pregnancy. Avoid the temptation of pouring through obstetric books to find out all the things that can go wrong!

The same goes for films. Helen Brew's film is probably best seen before you get pregnant, not in pregnancy, as it is shocking. 'Birth: a film about feelings and experiences' is fine for pregnancy. Some large hospitals, e.g. Queen Charlotte's, have their own birth films.

Some people may advise you to read one book only and stick to the ideas it presents, and may even say that if you read a good deal you will get 'confused'. This is ridiculous. Read as much as you feel you want to, but preferably not actually in labour.

Virginia Apgar and Joan Beck: *Is my baby all right?* Trident Press, New York (1972).
Suzanne Arms: *Immaculate deception,* Houghton Mifflers, Boston (1975).
Constance Bean: *Methods of childbirth,* Doubleday, New York (1972).
Elisabeth Bing: *Six practical lessons for an easier childbirth,* Bantam Books, New York (1969).
—— *The adventure of birth,* Simon & Schuster, New York (1970).
Boston Women's Health Book Collective: *Our bodies, ourselves,* Simon & Schuster, New York (1976).
—— *Ourselves and our children,* Random House, New York (1978).
Gordon Bourne: *Pregnancy,* Cassell, London, (1972), (Pan revised edition 1975; Harper & Row, New York 1974).
Herbert and Margaret Brant: *Dictionary of pregnancy, childbirth and contraception,* Mayflower, London (1971).
Danae Brook: *Naturebirth,* Penguin, Harmondsworth (1976).
Janet Brown and others: *Two births,* Random House, New York (1972).
E. Carway & Y. Brackbill: *Effects of obstetrical medication on the*

147

Bibliography

fetus and infant, Society for Research in Child Development, 35(1970).

Tim Chard and Martin Richards: *Benefits and hazards of the new obstetrics,* Spastics International Medical Publications, 1977. Heinemann, London (1977).

J. Chassar Moir: *Scientific foundations of obstetrics and gynaecology* (ed. Elliot Philipp, Josephine Barnes, and Michael Newton), Heinemann, London (1970).

Arthur D. and Libby L. Colman: *Pregnancy: the psychological experience,* Herder & Herder, New York (1972).

P. A. Davies, R. J. Robinson, J. W. Scopes, J. P. M. Tizard, and J. S. Wigglesworth: *Medical care of newborn babies,* Clinics in Developmental Medicine 44145, Heinemann, London (1972).

Grantly Dick Read: *Childbirth without fear,* Heinemann Medical, London (1942). (5th edition revised 1968, Harper & Row, New York 1970.)

Jean Donnison: *Midwives and medical men,* Heinemann, London (1977).

Barbara Ehrenreich and Deirdre English: *For her own good,* Anchor Press/Doubleday, New York (1978).

Valmai Howe Elkins: *The rights of the pregnant parent,* Waxwing Productions, Ottawa and Two Continents Publishing Group, New York (1976).

Donna and Roger Ewy: *Preparation for childbirth,* Pruett Publishing Co, Boulder, Colorado (1970). (Available through ICEA Supplies Center, PO Box 70258, Seattle, WA 98107, USA.)

Robert T. Francoeur: *Utopian motherhood,* George Allen & Unwin (1971).

D. Gardner and D. Hull (Eds.): *Recent advances in paediatrics,* Churchill, London (1971).

Ina May Gaskin: *Spiritual midwifery,* The Book Publishing Company, Tennessee (1978).

Alan F. Guttmacher: *Pregnancy and birth,* New American Library, New York (1971).

Doris Haire: *The cultural warping of childbirth,* ICEA Bookstore, PO Box 70258, Seattle WA 98107 (1972).

D. F. Hawkins (Ed.): *Obstetric therapeutics,* Bailliere Tindall, London (1974).

P. J. Huntingford, R. W. Beard, F. E. Hytten, and J. W. Scopes (Eds.): *Perinatal medicine,* Karger, Basel (1970).

Ivan Illich: *Medical nemesis,* Pantheon Books, London (1976).

Sheila Kitzinger: *The experience of childbirth,* Gollancz, London (1962). (Penguin, London 1967; 5th Penguin edition, London 1977; Taplinger, New York 1972; Penguin, New York 1972.)

—— *Giving Birth: The parents' emotions in childbirth,* 2nd Sphere edition, London 1979. (Sphere, London 1972; Taplinger, New York 1972; Schocken Books, New York 1978.)

Birth at home

—— *Some mothers' experiences of induced labour,* National Childbirth Trust, London 2nd ed. (1978)

—— Education and counselling for childbirth, Bailliere Tindall, London (1977). (Schocken, New York 1979.)

—— *Women as mothers,* Fontana, London (1978).

—— *The place of birth* (ed. with John Davis), Oxford University Press (1978).

—— *The good birth guide,* Fontana, London (1979).

—— *Journey through birth* (a set of cassette tape recordings). Julian Aston Productions, London and New York (1976).

Marshall H. Klaus and John H. Kennell: *Maternal – infant bonding,* Mosby, St. Louis (1976).

Raven Lang: *The birth book,* Genesis Press, Calif. (1972).

Penelope Leach: *Baby and child,* Michael Joseph, London (1977).

Frédérick Leboyer: *Birth without violence,* Fontana, London (1977).

Derek Llewellyn-Jones: *Fundamentals of obstetrics and gynaecology,* Vol. 1; *Obstetrics,* Faber, London (1973).

—— *Everywoman,* Faber, London (1971).

Aidan Macfarlane: *The psychology of childbirth,* Fontana, London (1977).

Elliott H. McCleary: *New miracles of childbirth,* McKay, New York (1974).

Nancy MacKeith: *Women's health handbook,* Virago, London (1978).

Caterine Milinaire: *Birth,* Harmony Books, New York, (1974).

D. D. Moir: *Pain relief in labour,* Churchill Livingstone, Edinburgh (1941).

Margaret Myles: *Textbook for midwives,* Churchill Livingstone, Edinburgh (1972).

National Birthday Trust and Royal College of Obstetrics and Gynaecology: *British Births 1970,* Vol. 1: *The first week of life,* Heinemann, London (1975); Vol. II: Obstetric Care (1978)

Rebecca Rowe Parfitt: *The birth primer,* Running Press, Philadelphia (1977).

Elliot Philipp: *Childbirth,* Fontana, London (1978).

Angela Phillips and Jill Rakusen: *Our bodies ourselves,* Penguin, Harmondsworth (1978).

Rudolph Schaffer: *Mothering,* Fontana, London (1977).

Marion Sousa: *Childbirth at home,* Bantam, New York (1977).

Nancy Stoller Shaw: *Forced labor,* Pergamon Press, New York (1974).

David and Lee Stewart (Eds.): *Safe alternatives in childbirth,* NAPSAC, Chapel Hill, North Carolina (1976).

Deborah Tanzer and Jean Block: *Why natural childbirth?* Doubleday, New York (1972).

Polly Toynbee: *Hospital (chapter on birth),* Hutchinson, London (1977).

Bibliography

Films

The First Days of Life with Pierre Vellay, Boulter Hawke Films, Suffolk. Can be hired.

Birth: A film about feelings and experiences with Sheila Kitzinger and Frédérick Leboyer. Producer Julian Aston; can be hired from The Birth Centre, 188 Old Street, London E.C.1.

Birth. Producer Helen Brew. With R. D. Laing. Can be hired from Concorde Film Council, 201 Felixstowe Road, Ipswich, Suffolk.

Open University course: *The first years of life,* Apply Open University, Milton Keynes, Bucks. There is special course material on birth.

Index

Index

Index

Index